Home Remedies

D1642777

Otto Wolff

Home Remedies

Herbal and homeopathic
treatments for use at home

Translated by A.R. Meuss and J. Collis

Floris Books

Originally published in German as *Die naturgemässe Haus-apotheke* by Verlag Freies Geistesleben, Stuttgart, 1988.
First published in English by Floris Books, Edinburgh, 1991.
Revised edition published in 2000.

British Library CIP data available

ISBN 0–86315–319–4

Printed in Great Britain by
J W Arrowsmith, Bristol

Contents

Preface

The aim of this book is to give practical advice on how to deal with health problems using natural methods. Information on the use of conventional drugs and methods is easily available with many books on the subject. Painkillers, sleeping pills, sedatives, laxatives and so on are widely used nowadays and most people are familiar with them; all the information for their use is given on the packs or enclosed leaflets.

The sale of such medicines is increasing, a clear sign that they are effective — otherwise people would not buy them. But they offer only temporary relief from the problem and therefore have to be taken frequently or even continuously. As a result, sufferers then tend to think that they can no longer manage without the tablets, or they simply do not want to do without them, seeing that they offer such easy and rapid relief. With this attitude, some degree of drug dependence is taken for granted, along with side effects, and people fail to realize that the fundamental causes of the disorder have not been tackled at all.

Most of the drugs just mentioned are effective because they remove symptoms — that is, specific changes in the body indicating that something is wrong. For example, pain is removed with a painkiller. Other drugs replace a missing or inadequate function, typical examples being the use of enzymes to help digestion, and hormone replacement. While treatment of this kind is clearly necessary at times, it is important to remember that unpleasant symptoms like a temperature or pain can be signs warning us, for example, that we are overdoing things. Here, our bodily reactions are intended to force us to take a much-needed rest and can also help us to deal with more deep-seated problems.

This book aims to show ways in which biological and therefore natural methods can be used to resolve rather than suppress a pathological reaction. Treatment of this kind is designed not simply to deal with symptoms but to mobilize the whole body and its powers of self-healing.

Pain may have many causes. A painkiller will relieve any kind of pain, whatever its origin, and that may be considered an advantage. It acts rapidly, but on the other hand it does not treat the cause as such. True healing comes when the disease is resolved and overcome; this is more of an effort and also takes longer, for it is a process that must be initiated by the body itself.

The approach described in this book is based on the teachings of Rudolf Steiner (1861–1925), the founder of anthroposophy. This approach considers the human being as a whole, made up of body, soul and spirit, in relationship to the kingdoms of nature, using methods that are wholly in accord with modern thinking. Suggestions for further reading on this subject are given at the back of the book.

Steiner's insights provide a new understanding of many tried and tested old methods that are in tune with the world of nature and the human being. Medicinal baths, packs, compresses and special diets come under this heading as well as a number of medicaments. The latter derive mainly from plants, which from ancient times were felt instinctively to be a source of natural healing powers. The natural materials are frequently prepared as decimal potencies, using the method of homeopathy developed by Dr Samuel Hahnemann (1755–1843). This consists of a rhythmical sequence of 'dilution' and forceful agitation of the original material so that a point is reached where toxic effects have disappeared and the special powers of the substance are ac-

tivated. Medicines prepared in this way are generally prescribed on the basis of what is known as the 'homeopathic
drug picture,' produced by testing the medicine on healthy
human subjects. 'Drug tests on humans create a field of activity similar to that created by a disease. A drug capable of
producing such a combination of reactions can, if suitably
prepared, cure the same combination when it has been produced by disease.' This Law of Similars is the basis of homeopathy. Unfortunately homeopathy has barely found
acceptance in conventional medicine, much to the disad-
vantage of patients. 'Its undoubted successes ... are considered unacceptable because they have not been subject to
large-scale statistical analysis.' (Lockie 1989)

It should be noted, however, that successful homeopathic treatment calls for detailed knowledge of what specialists in the field call the 'drug pictures,' and the
standards that apply are very different from those used in
ordinary diagnosis. This means that different patients with
the 'same' disease may require different homeopathic medicines; conversely the same medicine may be prescribed
for a wide range of different diseases. Effective prescribing
calls for both knowledge and experience.

The advice given in this book is intended to help lay
people to deal with both minor illnesses and chronic conditions. The aim is not to make consulting your doctor unnecessary but to provide effective support. Non-medical
methods will also often help to improve things (hydrotherapy, for example, or diet), and these are also described in
the opening section. In no way does this mean that they are
all that is required, or that readers should in every case treat
themselves. **In all cases of serious or persistent illness, a
doctor should be consulted.**

Medicines

All the medicines referred to in the main body of the book
are listed at the back. Unless labelled POM (Prescription
Only Medicine), these do not require a prescription. They
may be obtained from homeopathic pharmacies, health
food stores or from local chemists, who will normally
order any that they do not have in stock. Homeopathic
medicines based on a single substance are sold as liquids
(drops, dilutions), in powder form (triturations), or as
tablets or pilules (globuli). As referred to above, the substances can be prepared to different potencies, being diluted many times and subjected to rhythmical shaking at
every dilution stage. The prepared substance is, where rel-
evant, designated with a number, for instance, Arnica 6 or
Arnica 30. The higher the number, the higher the potency.
In this book, the potency number is followed by an x so, for
example, Belladonna 3x indicates the third decimal potency of Belladonna, that is, the original substance diluted
1:10 three times.

It is important to note that just because a medicine is
available without prescription, it does not automatically
mean that it is harmless. The decision as to whether a medicine should be available with or without prescription may
in some areas be made by authorities whose experience is
in conventional medicine, where synthetic drugs are generally used, and who are usually sceptical when it comes to
natural medicine. Many of the painkillers sold over the
counter today contain paracetamol, for instance, a chemical compound that does not occur in nature. Long-term use
may cause liver damage and prove fatal. In spite of this,
tablets containing paracetamol are available without prescription.

On the other hand, some homeopathic medicines, for instance those that contain Belladonna 3x, may be available on prescription only, despite the fact that the risk of poisoning is practically nil at this low concentration and long-term use has not been found to cause damage. In some areas, preparations of Aristolochia (birthwort) are not available below the tenth potency, as cancer was observed in tests with animals subjected to a concentrate derived from the plant. In cases where inexpert use may indeed cause damage, it is of course quite right that some medicines should only be available on prescription.

A limited list of manufacturers is given in the Appendix to help with obtaining preparations or products; the mention of particular firms implies no specific approval. A full list of medicines referred to in this book is also provided. The symbol ® against the name of a medicine in the Appendix indicates that it is a registered name, that is, a specialty that has been patented.

For further background information and practical guidance, see the works listed under *Further Reading* at the back of the book.

Health and Illness

Nowadays people tend to go and see their doctor as soon as they feel off colour or notice anything wrong. In our fast-living world, patients often put pressure on their doctor to prescribe fast-acting drugs: they have appointments to keep, deadlines to meet, and do not want to miss out on anything. This is quite typical of attitudes towards medicine today — illness is seen as a spanner in the works and the doctor as a kind of mechanic who will find an instant cure for the problem. Mainly because of our whole attitude to life, there is practically no feeling left for the meaning of illness.

If we look upon the human being merely as a complex chemical and physical system, we are bound to regard illness as a technical defect that can be corrected by using the right chemical implement. Certainly, many problems can be dealt with in this way, but this does not mean that health has been restored. People often feel off colour for months after rapid recovery from a serious illness. Even the most thorough examination will fail to show anything wrong, and the individual concerned will be given tranquillizers or may be written off as a difficult patient, or just a complaining type. But the truth is that the absence of detectable symptoms does not automatically indicate a state of health.

Health is not a matter of the physical body alone, and if health care is to be truly comprehensive, it cannot be limited to the physical side, as is so often the case today; soul and spirit must also be taken into account.

We pay great attention in modern society to our physical well-being. The basic rules of hygiene, cleanliness and so on are generally known, and this is certainly a positive factor. Yet people have rather confused notions when it comes to healthy eating, sport, exercise and toughening the body, ideas that are generally taken from technology or chemistry. Such a viewpoint, however, is far from adequate where the human being is concerned, as the following discussion shows.

'Soul hygiene' is practically unknown today; compared to physical hygiene it counts really for nothing compared to, for example, the amount of time and money spent on sport or cosmetics. Illness, though, is a problem in soul and spirit that takes time, sometimes decades, before it manifests itself at the physical level.

In earlier times, soul hygiene was much more of a daily routine for people than physical hygiene. Thus the day would start and end with a prayer, and grace before meals came naturally. Today, many people no longer feel able to do this; life often seems to run at a more superficial level. To gain depth, we have to be capable of veneration and wonder. Modern people are no longer able to marvel at things but immediately ask for a scientific explanation. At most they will marvel at 'how far we have advanced' — Goethe poked fun at this in his *Faust*. Human achievements are still admired, but not creation or the wonders that we see in the world of nature. In reality every daisy, and indeed every blade of grass, is a marvel, something even the most advanced technology cannot create. From the very beginning, humanity recognized the life-creative powers as sublime spirits, referring to them as 'god' or 'gods.' When science and materialism became dominant, these higher powers were denied existence and people were told that everything had a scientific explanation based on the laws of physics and chemistry, on heredity, the principle of selection, chance, and so on, and that there was no need to assume the existence of higher forms of being. The result is the one-sided, limited image we have of the world today, cut off from its divine origins. Such a relationship to the world, with no morality and without meaning, must, in the long run, have a destructive effect on human beings and their environment.

The depth of our experience is also limited by endless stimulation of the senses. The images which flood out of advertising signs, illustrated magazines and television blanket the finer feelings that arise in the soul. The same applies to the constant background noise to which people are exposed — usually by choice — and which, unlike visual stimuli, cannot be escaped. Thus modern life stuns and distorts our inner life.*

Wonder is only felt by those capable of experiencing it. This means that we have to be open to beauty, to the experience of harmony and to true art. Soul hygiene can be positively practised by actively taking up any form of art (see *Further Reading* at the back of this book). If this proves impossible, it is important at least to take a living interest in classical works of art — reading poetry and prose, looking at paintings and other works of art or listening to classical music. What matters is not to register or analyse those works, but to come to inner experience, a positive response in heart and mind. The same can be achieved by looking at the world of nature. Again, it does not matter if we are unable to put names to the plants and animals; we need to develop a feeling for their way of life, the essence of their being, so that in perceiving the scent of a flower we also perceive the way the whole plant grows, or come to feel the

* For a discussion of problems related to modern life (the influence of television, pop music, etc.), see Treichler, *Soulways*.

pleasure and pain that exists in the sounds that animals make.

Hygiene of the spirit is something to which we give little thought these days. It is spirit that differentiates human beings from animals, for it is the immortal core of our being. If people are convinced that human beings are merely intelligent mammals, 'naked apes,' their whole life will take its orientation from this and be no more than the life of an intelligent animal. Instead, we should be able to control our animal nature and learn to guide it. Drives, passions, lack of inhibition and so on, are animal traits that estrange human beings from their true nature. This does not mean, of course, that such traits should be suppressed or eradicated. They need to be channelled in the right direction and transformed. This has profound practical implications for the whole of our lifestyle.

If, for example, we base our life on the principle of 'survival of the fittest,' the 'struggle for existence' and the accepted idea of natural selection, then the profit motive, ambition, desire for power and the lack of consideration, that go with it, will be the consciously or unconsciously desired goal, often dressed up in terms such as 'success' and 'efficiency.' The inhumanity of these qualities has consequences we know all too well in modern life; we all know what it is like to be rushed and under pressure, or caught up in the work process. In the final instance there is a total inability to relax. The whole of the modern 'civilized' world is subject to this. Years or decades of this lifestyle result in states ranging from anxiety, sleeplessness, nervousness and psychological problems to muscular and vascular spasm and all kinds of circulatory disorders.

Stress is a widely used term today and its effects have been studied in detail. It is, however, a different problem to limit stress; to recognize the destructive nature of the many unnecessary stimuli that flood the senses and stop them, so that periods of peace and quiet can restore the organism.

Fear is a less well-known factor in causing disease. 'Paralysed with fear' is a term we should take seriously. Fear paralyses the immune system. Yet fear and anxiety exist all over the world today. People are afraid of cancer, AIDS, bacteria, viruses, obesity, cholesterol, war, losing their money, youth and jobs — the list is endless. In many cases our anxieties are perfectly understandable, for instance if we have to face an opponent who is much bigger and stronger than we are. However, we have to realize that many of our fears are consciously or unconsciously kept artificially alive by the negative emphasis used in reporting. If this feeling of fear or anxiety persists for some time, it must inevitably lead to hopelessness, and hence helplessness and a feeling of powerlessness.

Yet how can we resist opposition that is so much stronger? In the first place we can see that many of these supposed dangers do not exist for the individual concerned, or are greatly exaggerated. Then we must understand that we need inner strength, or at least the courage to develop it. Just as fear weakens the immune system, so inner activity and positivity can strengthen it. This inner activity is the opposite of passive waiting and the desire for luck without effort which characterizes much of our life today (for instance gambling, speculation or lottery). This strength can be achieved by structured practice, but such practising is strenuous, and nowadays we try to avoid strain.

In our experience, what is more important than avoiding or battling against negativity, is the deliberate creating and practising of positivity. Part of this practice is, for instance, having adequate physical exercise as a balance to predominantly sedentary intellectual activity, though one must also be aware that physical training after a certain age can lead to a hardening and obstruction of mental activity.

Such inner activity will not be achieved through escapism, a rush of enthusiasm or whatever, but is developed through little things, like observing the blossoming of a flower, the stages of development of a young child, or contemplating art, which then brings deep joy and satisfaction.

Against this approach to life, we can set another that is best expressed in the words of the German poet, Goethe: 'Let human beings be noble-minded, good and kind, for this alone distinguishes them from all other life-forms known on earth.' These are truly human qualities that do not take their orientation from animal nature. But who teaches such virtues today, or practises them?

There is another area where our attitude to things of the spirit is of crucial importance. It makes a difference, for example, whether we consider someone who has died as having ceased to exist, or as someone who is now in the world of the spirit. The latter is the true state of affairs, but can, of course, only mean something to those who accept the reality of the spirit.

Many deeper human problems, which may manifest themselves as physical problems, are today due to the fact that people feel an inner emptiness, and experience life as meaningless; with the whole of existence cast in doubt, they may even contemplate suicide. Boredom and the wrong mental attitudes that result from it are common, particularly in the 'civilized' world, and there can be no doubt that these are pathological states. The only way of overcoming these dangers is to gain, first of all, a clear understanding of the ways in which body, soul and spirit relate to one another. To speak of 'health' only with regard to the body, leaving aside soul and spirit, amounts to regarding the body as a machine. Human health is not a fixed state; it is based on a constantly changing equilibrium that has to be achieved and maintained over and over again.

In the Western world there is a sharp increase in chronic

fatigue syndrome, which is puzzling for doctors. No organic damage is evident, and only sometimes is a viral infection present (Epstein-Barr). Nevertheless, this fatigue can lead to the inability to work. In a nutshell this is a case of the exhaustion of the life forces, and can be caused by an ongoing unhealthy diet, chronic poisoning, or even a 'blockage' caused by an infection in the teeth, tonsils or elsewhere. In most cases the liver suffers as it is respoinsible for enlivening the whole organism. While the liver is not actually ill, it is disturbed. For that reason a change in diet, as well as treatment of the liver can be helpful. In addition, warm or hot baths (sauna) can improve the condition. Medicines on their own have little effect.

Keeping healthy

'Medical treatment' is widely thought (and expected) to consist of the doctor doing little more than prescribing some medicine or other. But even the best medicines should be part of a wider and comprehensive treatment which addresses the whole individual. Indeed, doctors themselves speak of disease 'management,' and the whole range of possible treatment includes a wide variety of techniques in which the patient is looked on as a whole: massage, manipulation, baths, dietary measures, general counselling, and so on.

Chronic diseases, a problem of our age, are hardly ever cured with tablets only. The causes often go back years, decades or more, or are congenital or hereditary. We can really only say that a disease has been cured when the causes have been dealt with and are no longer operative.

Of course, it is not possible in every case to establish the specific cause of an illness, and yet certain types of cause

are perfectly apparent and still not recognized. It is generally accepted today, that physical illnesses may have psychological causes and are therefore unlikely to respond to
treatment given at the physical level only. There can be no
doubt that in these cases a change has to be made in the
way the individuals concerned respond at a deeper level.

All too often, the spiritual background of illness is disregarded. We have discussed how an approach to life that
ignores the full nature of man can lead to illness. In some
cases special measures will be needed. Words can wound
and, in the same way, words spoken from the heart can also
heal. Above all, we must recognize the need to nurture the
life of soul and spirit.

Many of the diseases of our time involve the metabolic
system. The most obvious cause to be looked for is in the
food we eat and its effect on metabolism. Apart from the
need to nurture soul and spirit, the main steps to a healthy
life are through nutrition, the effective use of baths and
physical exercise (training), and these are discussed below.

Healthy eating

Only the broad outlines of this topic can be discussed here,
and there are many books which go into more detail on the
subject (see *Further Reading* at the back of this book). Certain aspects of our modern eating habits are quite likely to
make people ill or prevent them from getting well. In general terms, we can say of modern dietary habits that:
— we eat too much;
— our meals generally contain too much fat and protein;
— many foods are grown and processed in the wrong way;
— meals tend to be unbalanced;
— methods of preparing and cooking food are often inappropriate.

Prosperity has brought diseases that were formerly unknown and which affect above all the liver, gall-bladder and stomach, that is, the metabolic system; another group is made up of diseases where crystalline deposits are formed. The old rules, 'Don't eat unless you're hungry' and 'Stop eating when you're enjoying it most' are still valid for our health today. Continuing to eat when we are no longer hungry is a form of self-indulgence that can of course be enhanced by all kinds of culinary refinements. The healthy approach is not to forgo all enjoyment but to eat in moderation.

In the past, 'good' food meant 'rich' food. Meals with a high fat content do indeed keep us feeling satisfied for longer. 'Rich' people are 'satisfied' people. The poor, especially in times of need, traditionally lacked adequate fat in their diet. Today, fats are cheap and freely available, and because of this our diet tends to contain too much fat, most of it in the form of margarine and similar products that are much cheaper than butter. Most margarines contain oil and chemically hardened fats and therefore lack organic wholeness. Butter on the other hand comes from a living organism, and can be shown to have the universal character that a growing organism needs right down to its chemical structure.

The value of protein is overrated nowadays, and egg and meat consumption has steadily increased in recent decades. The consequence for many people is that the metabolism is overburdened, particularly on the acid side, which leads to chronic inflammation or increased toxic waste products in the body. Pork presents particular problems; those with rheumatic conditions will often note aggravation the day after they have eaten pork or pork products. Ancient Jewish and Muslim culture had a natural feeling for this, and eating pork was forbidden. In recent years, pork production has steadily increased and the consequences for general health, particularly for those with metabolic problems, cannot be foreseen. For most people, a change to a low-meat or vegetarian diet will reduce the burden on the organism and improve health.

It is important to differentiate between types of fat or protein. Olive oil, butter, and so on, are quite different kinds of fat; eggs, cheese and chicken are different sources of protein; and so on. Equally, we cannot look upon all carbohydrates as the same; we must distinguish between vegetables, potatoes, rice, sugar, and so on, all of which have quite different effects on the human being.

The closer that foods are to life, the fresher and less processed they are, the more 'life' they contain, which is what really matters. Refined foods such as white sugar and flour and products made with these are practically dead. Their 'life' has been removed, which makes them keep longer and offers other practical 'advantages;' biologically, however, that is, in terms of real value to life, they are almost worthless. They are of course easily digestible and provide instant 'energy' (glucose, for example), but that is not life. Quite the contrary, 'empty' carbohydrates of this kind — having practically no vitamins or minerals — actually deprive us of vitality, though this is not immediately apparent. One cannot deny that these products tend to taste delicious, as taste not only relates to quality but also provides enjoyment. But enjoyment does not equate with quality. Of course, we should enjoy the things that life has to offer, but if enjoyment comes to be seen as the only purpose of taking food we are headed for disaster: excessive weight or some common metabolic disorder will be the price we have to pay.

Food production is nowadays largely governed by the profit motive, with little regard for the biological needs of plants and animals. It goes without saying that the meat of chickens who have never seen natural light, a grain of corn or even a blade of grass, cannot be of good biological quality. The same applies to calves fed on dried milk and kept in the dark in order to produce white veal. Apples and vegetables can owe their perfect appearance to applications of chemical sprays. The risk to health comes not only from residues of these far from safe chemicals but also from the poor biological quality that those treatments hide. Tinned and bottled foods and preserves are more for emergencies or occasional convenience; they are not fit to make up a whole diet or for long-term use. Really fresh food has lots of vitality and should be a constituent of every meal. Raw food diets should be reserved for therapeutic purposes.

Biodynamic agriculture is based on the biological needs of plants and animals. Its products, marketed under the Demeter label, have been grown in healthy conditions that start with the soil.* Foods are specially prepared to make them more digestible and tasty, mainly using gentle heat to steam, braise, boil, roast or fry food. The method is chosen according to the nature of the food. If the process goes too far (boiling things to death), the vitality of food is destroyed.

Apart from general rules for healthy eating, individual needs also have to be taken into account. Meat or salt may be right for one person and wrong for another. Many people do not tolerate certain foods, which may indicate either organic weakness or that foods have been wrongly combined. In some cases, the problem can be quite narrowly specified. This is where the professional skills of a trained dietitian are needed.

Another factor is the time of the main meal, and skipping lunch. Research has shown that the same nutrients work differently in the morning from the evening. A sweet breakfast goes against the natural rhythm of the liver.

* For further reading see the section on 'Basic nutrition and biodynamic farming' (p.122).

Furthermore experiments on volunteers have shown that a large breakfast has little effect on body weight, while a large evening meal does.

We must not forget the real reason why we need food. It is not just a matter of taking in calories equivalent to a certain amount of heat energy, but of stimulating life, which only 'living' food can do. The right food is therefore a real life support, provided it retains a high degree of vitality and as little of this as possible is lost in preparation. In past times, food was felt to be the gift of heaven or of a divine world; grace at meals was a way of expressing gratitude for this gift. Even today, people cannot really live healthy lives unless they develop the right attitude to their food.

Therapeutic use of water and baths

Applications of hot and cold water are an ancient form of treatment. Some medicinal springs have been famed for centuries for virtues that depend not entirely on their chemical composition. Hydrotherapy, developed in modern times to become an indispensable part of natural medicine, can be practised at home with very beneficial effects. The founders of hydrotherapy were able to cure many patients — including many with serious illnesses — using external applications of water, a method much undervalued in an age where medicine is thought to consist mainly of taking pills.

Cold water applications
Some of the ground rules for applications of cold water are listed below. They are essential if the treatment is to be health-giving.

1   the body must be warm before cold applications are
    made;
2   the colder the water, the shorter the application;
3   it is the reaction to the cold water application that mat-
    ters; that is, the part of the body to which application
    was made should get warm after a while. This is
    achieved by getting into a warm bed after the treatment
    or getting the feet warm, for instance, by walking.

Hydrotherapy is primarily a form of vascular training, but
it also exercises the heat organism. Everything said in the
section on exercise therefore applies in this case as well.
Hydrotherapy is particularly beneficial for people who are
sensitive to cold. In practice, one starts with short, weak
stimuli, increasing both strength and duration day by day.
Many sensitivities can be overcome in this way.

Alternating hot and cold baths

As cold applications should only be made to parts that are
warm, cold feet for example are treated with alternating hot
and cold baths. Fill two footbaths or buckets with water:
one with water at a temperature of 37–39°C (99–102°F),
the other with tap water (about 15–20°C, 59–68°F). The
limb is first immersed in the warm water (about two minutes), then in the cold (twenty seconds to one minute), and
this is repeated several times, finishing with the warm
water. This is an excellent form of vascular training and
particularly effective at night, for instance to treat sleeplessness due to circulatory disorders. Anyone with consti-
tutionally cold feet should take care to put on clean socks
every day as well.

    Alternating hot and cold arm baths are highly effective
vascular training for the circulation of the heart in cases of
angina.

    The 'derivative action of water' (that is, drawing off the

disease process) is due to the fact that the application is made to a part of the body that is not affected by the disease. It is possible, for example, to treat congestion of blood in the head with a cold water affusion (pouring water over a part) applied to the calves of the legs; this restores a balanced circulation. The vascular training achieved by water applications of this kind has a stimulant effect on the whole body and can have a positive effect on chronic headaches and all kinds of circulatory disorders.

Using cold water treatments in conjunction with a prescribed diet and lifestyle designed to detoxicate the organism, the founders of hydrotherapy achieved remarkable results in the treatment of chronic diseases.

Hot water applications

Hot water applications are an entirely different story. Essentially they are used to achieve a rapid warming effect. For instance, if the body has got chilled through, the organism will usually produce additional heat after some time to counteract this, that is, the individual gets a temperature. The popular way of describing this is to say 'I've got a cold,' which is absolutely correct. Officially this is called an 'infection' nowadays, but it is not really the bacterial or viral infection that gives us a cold. These organisms only find a suitable soil in which to grow and multiply if the organism has been weakened and made receptive, for instance by getting chilled. The practical conclusion to be drawn is that a chill can be counteracted by a hot bath, and this will prevent the temperature and 'infection.' Please note that sweat baths are no longer suitable if the body temperature is already rising.

Sweat baths thoroughly warm the body and at the same time encourage sweating and therefore elimination of waste products via the skin. The method is to start at 37°C

(99°F), gradually increasing to 38.5°C (101°F), staying at that temperature for 5–10 minutes. Then hot water is added to bring the temperature quickly to 40–41°C (104–106°F) or even more. At this point the patient starts to sweat, is wrapped in a bath towel but not dried and put to bed to complete the sweating process. Caution is indicated with people who have a weak circulation; in their case water temperatures as high as 40–41°C (104–106°F) should be avoided. Instead, a cloth soaked in cold water is placed on the forehead, and Cardiodoron A is given before the bath, three applications of 10–15 drops at ten to twenty minute intervals. It is clearly not advisable to have a bath on a full stomach, and it is a good idea to go to the lavatory before-hand.

Saunas serve a similar function to sweat baths, with the cold plunge that follows also providing vascular training.

Hyperthermal baths (developed by the Austrian Maria Schlenz) use relatively high water temperatures, so that the body temperature may be above 40°C (104°F) for limited periods. They should only be given by trained personnel, for they represent a major intervention in the composition of the organism — with, of course, correspondingly high healing potential.

A milder form of detoxication is achieved with a **soap bath**. Thoroughly soap the whole body during a bath, leave to act for some minutes and rinse well.

Soda baths have a similar effect. Add a handful of soda crystals to the water; water temperature 37–38°C (99–100°F), duration about twenty minutes. They are also a useful preventive method against a number of virus infections such as influenza.

For a **rosemary bath**, add about a tablespoonful of Rosemary Bath Milk to the bath.

Lavender baths are soothing and calming and particularly helpful in cases of sleeplessness, nervousness and nervous diseases. Water temperature 36–37°C (97–99°F).

Oil dispersion baths need a special apparatus that creates a very fine dispersion of oil in water. This makes it easier for medicinal substances added to the water to be absorbed through the skin. These baths stimulate the internal warmth processes, thus activating the warmth organism, rather than passively increasing the warmth. Therefore the bath should have a temperature of only 36°C (97°F). During subsequent rest in bed this inner warmth is developed. This is a vital element in the treatment of most chronic illnesses, particularly circulatory problems. Different oils are used depending on the type of disorder.

Exercise

Physical exercises can be used to strengthen particular organs or their function. Regular exercise will increase performance levels. It is important not to overdo this but make exercises harder and longer gradually, which calls for perseverance. Excessive physical demands cause poisoning with metabolic waste products resulting in, for example, muscle pain felt after excessive exercise, which means temporary damage to muscle tissues. There are however lower limits, too. An exercise carried out with too little effort or done for too short a time will not enhance performance. What matters most of all is that exercise is done regularly.

Physical training is generally considered as a form of sport. While this has a good side, it can also bring the desire to improve 'performance' in a specialized area. Narrowly focused efforts of this kind have nothing to do with improving health. The sort of super-performance that we

see in top athletes almost inevitably implies over-special-
ization and physical strain and even muscle spasms. Anyone active in sport for the sake of their health should not try
to emulate top athletes, who are specialists, but should take
their exercise in a variety of forms, such as walking and
swimming.

To conclude we can observe that many man-made envi-
ronmental influences can be as damaging to health as a
spirit-denying attitude to life. It is up to each individual to
understand these influences, to avoid them where possible,
perhaps even to do without some conveniences in order to
find a more positive lifestyle.

General Health Problems

Pain

Pain is a warning sign and not a disease (see p.9f). Getting rid of pain therefore in no way represents a cure. It may however be necessary to give pain relief, using one of the many painkillers now on the market if the pain is extremely severe. On the other hand it is sometimes possible to relieve pain completely or at least partly by using very simple methods. Heat will often help, particularly with colics. Conversely, some types of headache respond to the application of cold (ice bag).

Petasites e rad. is universally effective in relieving tension pain (25 mg capsules). Essential oils have general relaxing and sedative properties and are particularly useful in support of heat applications. The best method is to put a few drops on a hot compress that is applied locally, or massage them gently into the affected area. Japanese Peppermint Oil is one of the oils to be used for this purpose, or combinations of oils such as Olbas Oil and Melissa comp.

Colicky and spastic pain in the abdomen may respond to a combination of Belladonna 4x and Podophyllum 4x (10 drops several times a day).

For neuralgia, see p.52.

Injuries (trauma)

In general, healing is generally stimulated by taking Arnica 3x, 5–7 drops initially at hourly intervals and after some days 10 drops three times a day.

Cuts, open wounds

Stitches or clips to close the wound should be applied by a doctor. The edges of smaller wounds can be brought together with a first aid dressing and the wound left to dry.

Abrasions

Cover thickly with WCS Powder and a non-adhesive dressing or emergency dressing.

Infected wounds

Compresses with Calendula Lotion, a tablespoonful to a cup of lukewarm water; renew about every four hours. Dressings with Weleda Balsamicum Ointment or Mercurialis comp. ointment. Dressings with Weleda Wound Healing Ointment or Peru-Lenicet Ointment.

Contusions, bruises, haematomas

As soon as possible apply compresses with Arnica Lotion (a teaspoonful to a cup of lukewarm water). Later apply Arnica Ointment until healing is complete.

Strains, sprains, torn ligaments

Immediately apply an elastic bandage firmly, loosening it after one or two hours. In case of dislocations and torn ligaments consult a doctor.

Immediately after the accident, apply Arnica Lotion (see above). Potters Comfrey Ointment is beneficial later on.

The joint needs to be strapped for at least four to six weeks and also later if subjected to weight, stress or strain.

Fractures slow to heal

Fractures are sometimes slow to unite. Healing is stimulated by giving Arnica 3x, 10 drops at hourly intervals to begin with, changing to 15 drops three times daily after three days, and after about a week, Weleda Calcium Supplement 1 and 2 (No. 1 in the mornings, No. 2 at night), a good pinch of powder or 1 tablet. Preparations based on Comfrey (Symphytum) are also indicated.

Burns

Never use flour, oil, powders, talc, or anything like these. Immediately put the burned part into clean cold water; ordinary tap water is perfectly good for the purpose. This will not only relieve the pain but also help to dissolve out the toxic products that have formed. Subsequent healing will be much better than if ointments or powders have been used. Add Combudoron Lotion 1:10, that is, 100 ml to a litre (4 fl oz to a quart) of water (even better, to water containing just under 1% of common salt). Renew the liquid every six hours. If total immersion of the part is not possible, put thick layers of gauze soaked in cold diluted Combudoron Lotion on the burn; keep moist all the time by trickling on more of the liquid. Renew the gauze every 6–8 hours. If blisters form, do not cut them open but dab with alcohol and pierce with a sterilized needle, so that the fluid can run out.

Depending on the size of the area and the severity of the burn, patients may develop a severe general reaction and go into shock. This requires hospital treatment. Always give the patient (not if unconscious) water or tea to drink (never alcohol), ideally with some salt added.

When the wounds start to heal, treat with Combudoron Ointment.

Combudoron Gel is particularly useful for treating burns in the face and sunburn. Apply thickly.

Insect bites

Dab with undiluted Combudoron Lotion or apply Combudoron Gel.

Weather, sensitivity to changes

Solum oliginosum comp. is beneficial. Take 10–15 pilules several times daily. Sometimes the same preparation acts better as a bath, with 2 tablespoons of the Bath Lotion added to a full bath. In very severe cases it may be given by injection under medical supervision.

Travel problems

Travel sickness

Nausea and vomiting in conjunction with circulatory insufficiency may develop due to the rocking movement experienced when travelling by boat, plane or car.

Travel sickness pills designed to relieve the symptoms do not offer a long-term solution and have to be taken again on every occasion. It is therefore better to address the underlying sensitivity. One method is to take Nausyn, 5–8 drops or 1 or 2 tablets three to five times daily for two or three weeks before starting the journey. This will usually prevent the symptoms from developing.

A simple method that often proves effective is to be mentally involved in the job of driving the vehicle even as a passenger. It is well known, for example, that some people only get car-sick as passengers but not when they drive themselves.

Gastrointestinal problems

Air travel means that people often find themselves trans-
ported to a completely different climate, lifestyle and diet
within hours. Both acute and chronic illnesses may result.

Moving from a cooler to a hotter climate frequently results in gastroenteritis. The causes are many and varied,
among them taking more frequent cold drinks. The body
loses fluids more rapidly in a hot climate and these have to
be replaced, but it is better not to take ice-cold drinks. Sensitive subjects should ask for warm, not hot, drinks. Sweating also means the loss of salts. The simplest way of
replacing both salt and liquids is to take plenty of soup.
Drinking after meals is particularly bad. Liquids taken
after a sweet dessert and particularly also after fruit, encourage fermentation. The best time for taking liquids is
between meals or up to twenty minutes before meals as an
aperitif.

Contaminated food, especially fruit, can be a source of
infection and cause severe diarrhoea. It is clearly a good
idea to wash fruit, but in the case of grapes or very soft fruit
such washing has mainly symbolic character, as it is unlikely to remove bacterial contamination and pesticide
residues. Apples, however, can be effectively cleaned.

The question is, why do some people get ill after eating
a particular food and others do not. This often has to do with
gastric acid, which not only aids digestion but also kills bacteria. Some people have too little gastric acid or even none
at all, and are therefore more susceptible. The most important thing is not to dilute what gastric acid there is by drinking just before meals (that is, twenty minutes or less before
eating). Good quality soup does of course also dilute the
acid, but it also stimulates the production of new gastric
acid. It is therefore a good idea to start a meal with soup.

The next step is to replace the missing gastric acid. A citrated pepsin mixture taken before meals will generally prevent 'tummy upsets' when abroad. Undiluted lemon juice is slightly less effective but on the other hand easy to obtain. It is best added to the food — which is what the locals generally do — and not taken in sweetened lemon drinks or lemonade.

Hepatitis

Hepatitis is easily picked up in hot countries and is a much more dangerous condition than a stomach upset or diarrhoea. The early symptoms are often mistaken for a stomach upset, loss of appetite, indigestion, a chill, and so on, but the diagnosis is immediately obvious if jaundice develops. This may not always happen, however. When gastrointestinal symptoms disappear but lack of appetite, tiredness and lack of drive persist, there is a strong suspicion that the 'upset stomach' was, or still is, hepatitis. A doctor should be consulted. The dietary measures listed on p.77f will also be required.

Some degree of protection from all the above disorders is achieved by careful hygiene, restraint in the choice and amount of foods and above all keeping warm. In the past, people would wear cummerbunds or body belts particularly in hot climates and so protect the liver, stomach and intestines from chills. This is still a sensible idea.

Jet lag

Fast travel from east to west, and even more so from west to east, creates its own problems. The time difference between Europe and North America, for instance, is six hours or more and the organism needs several days to adjust to this as the body rhythms have to adapt to different earth rhythms.

Cardiodoron A is beneficial in this situation. It acts on rhythmical processes in the body and particularly the cardiovascular system. Take 10 drops three times daily for two or three days before starting the journey, 10–15 drops several times daily during the journey, and the same dose for another two or three days after the journey.

Fever

A raised temperature is a common symptom of influenza and other infectious diseases. Fever is not an illness, but (as was known in the past) a meaningful reaction. Other symptoms are exhaustion, headaches and general malaise. People generally think it is a good idea to bring the temperature down as fast as possible, so that the patient feels better. The usual influenza remedies almost all contain anti-fever drugs. This method of treatment does, however, go against the body's efforts to heal itself. A temperature plays an important role in defending the organism against viruses and bacteria, so that it is not usually a good idea to suppress it. With natural medicine the aim is to work with the fever, limiting it if it gets too high and promoting a temperature if the body is unable to do it adequately for itself. By contrast, the most commonly used measures to bring down a temperature deprive the body of its most important weapon against bacteria and viruses. It is true that the acute symptoms disappear quite quickly, but recovery tends to be extremely slow and a chronic state of ill-health may develop or a 'syndrome shift' (a new disease taking the place of the old one that has not been fully over-come). Suppression also means failure to stimulate and strengthen the immune system.

If the immune system collapses completely, the way is open for cancer to develop. For some decades it has been known that cancer patients have no history of febrile ill-nesses and no childhood illnesses, but no one has thought of the long-term effects of suppression of fever after ten to thirty years.

Adequate detoxication is important for the whole time that the disease runs its course. Therefore it must be en-sured that the bowels are emptied (using a laxative tea or, for more rapid action, an enema), and, for as long as the pa-tient has a temperature, plenty of fluids are taken. Loss of appetite with a temperature is a protective measure on the part of the organism. Avoid all high-protein foods and eat as little as possible. Any loss of weight will soon be com-pensated following recovery.

If a cold is starting, or suspected to be starting, it is im-portant to get the body really warm. This is best achieved with a hot bath, sauna or other ways of producing a sweat, and by drinking lime blossom or elderflower tea. If the temperature is already rising, a hot bath or sauna are no longer suitable, but a sweat, herb teas and keeping the bow-els open are appropriate.

For febrile convulsions of children, see p.100.

Specific Conditions

Skin conditions

'The skin shows what is going on inside' is an old saying that every doctor was familiar with in the past. When we grow red with embarrassment or go pale with fright, our inner life is quite obviously reflected by the skin. The term 'skin eruption' is also highly expressive; 'eczema' and 'exanthema' are based on the Greek words for 'eruption' and 'breaking into flower.' Functional disorders of internal organs thus come to expression in the skin. A well-known instance is the alternation between certain types of skin eruption and liver disorders, with the eruption coming up when the liver seems to be 'in order' and conversely the liver and metabolism making themselves felt once the skin problem has gone. It calls for considerable medical skill to establish which organic function is upset with a particular skin condition, a task that is not merely difficult but sometimes quite impossible, as there are so many factors involved. The skin also protects us from external factors, and 'skin diseases' may be reactions to these, particularly if the individual has an allergy. Finally there are also skin problems that arise in the skin itself and do not depend on either internal or external factors.

Metabolic disorders are a common factor and therefore

make a good starting point. A balanced diet is of prime importance, though little attention is paid to this by most modern dermatologists. Too much protein — meat, and particularly pork — makes individuals more prone to develop inflammation and suppuration; four weeks on a raw food diet excluding proteins will overcome the problem. Salt makes the tissues hold water. Water retention and, above all, skin irritation will often respond instantly to a completely salt-free diet. Many foods (bread, cheese, particularly hard cheeses, fish and rich foods) contain large amounts of salt, and a completely salt-free diet is not easy to accept.

Some skin conditions are due to intolerance of certain foods, with milk and milk products frequently the culprits; omitting these (except for butter) will often give remarkable improvement. These are just a few examples of the many ways, far from fully explored as yet, in which diet can influence skin disease.

Eczema

In the case of **weeping eczema**, the rule still holds that wet (weeping) skin eruptions need wet treatment, for instance, lukewarm compresses with water to which Calendula Essence has been added. Compresses with oak bark decoctions will often dry lesions even more rapidly. Boil 2 or 3 tablespoons of the pure oak bark preparation briefly in 1 litre (quart) of water and use for compresses; renew compresses after thirty minutes. The fabric of the compress will stain brown and the stain will not wash out. Irritation is reduced by application of cod liver oil ointment or camomile ointment.

Some skins do not tolerate soap or alkaline washing agents. In this case, Lactisol, a product made from whey, may be added to the bath water or used in compresses; it restores the acid balance of the skin.

Weeping eruptions (also vesicular eruptions) are also helped by drinking Equisetum (horsetail) tea, which needs to be boiled, not just infused, or by taking Equisetum 4x or, with chronic conditions, 15x.

Dry eczema is generally treated with ointments. Oils tend to be drying, so that ointments with a partly aqueous base are preferable.

Chronic dry eczema clearly needs long-term treatment, including the right kind of diet (see above) and open bowels (see also under Constipation on p.73), that is, measures that influence general metabolism.

Calendula/Stibium ointment is the basic treatment for dry skin eruptions.

Acne

This is a metabolic disorder caused by hormone imbalance, which is why it is so common in puberty. Dietary measures include complete avoidance of chocolate, sweets, meat and eggs for some weeks. Little fat should be taken and hardened fats such as margarine avoided completely. Later, pork should still be avoided and sugar reduced to a minimum. A good method is a few weeks on a diet based on barley and millet, which may be prepared in all kinds of different ways. The skin should be washed with warm water, preferably boiled in advance, and sulphur soap.

Many preparations are available for external use, among them those based on ichthammol, a natural oil distilled from bituminous schist or shale, obtainable from pharmacies.

Internally, yeast preparations are helpful, the simplest being fresh baker's yeast.

Balanced combinations of external and internal treatments are also on the market, among them the Wala Acne Treatment.

Milk crust

A condition sometimes seen in babies. Often, but not always, intolerance of cow's milk is the reason, so that a change should be made to non-milk products (soya products, almond milk), at least for a time. Moist compresses with a tea made from wild pansy (Viola tricolor) are helpful. Internally give Dermatodoron, 5–10 drops three times daily.

Neurodermatitis

As the name suggests, many of the causes are to do with the nerves. This is a complex syndrome which also has an allergic element to it. It may thus follow milk crust or alternate with asthma. Ointments will give relief but cannot cure the condition. It is important to eliminate any allergen (often milk products, or also wheat) and above all also to reduce tension, which in the case of children means the parents have to be included. It needs real skill to find the right medication. Evening Primrose Oil, rich in specific unsaturated fatty acids (incl. gamma linolenic acid) helps to reduce the irritation. The capsules (e.g. Efamol) are taken by mouth.

Allergic skin eruptions

Eliminate the allergen that causes the condition. Consider a change in diet. Take care to keep the bowels open. Camomile ointment helps to reduce irritation.

Athlete's foot

Fungal infections may affect not only the toenails but also fingernails and skin. A vast number of fungicidal products are available, but these do not take account of the 'soil,' the conditions created in which the fungus is able to flourish. These arise when the structures that separate the internal world from the environment partly break down. Various fatty acids, also combined with iodine, provide tissue stimulation and protection. Preparations for external use include preparations containing ichthammol (see p.45, *Acne*).

Herpes labialis (cold sores)

Vesicles often develop on the lips when one has a temperature or virus infection. They are essentially harmless and will heal up in a few days.

If the sores come up more frequently and also when there is no temperature, they can be prevented by taking Cantharis 10x, about 7 drops every thirty minutes, as soon as there is the first indication of a sore developing. A 1% extract of Melissa (balm) may be used externally.

The head and nervous system

Headache

Frequent headaches need to have the cause established.
Depending on the given situation, it may sometimes be sufficient to relieve the strain on metabolism by clearing the
bowels, taking a footbath with rising water temperature, or
massage the back of the neck with Aconitum comp.,
Oleum.

Migraine

Migraine attacks generally take the form of severe
headache on one side of the head.

Attention should be given to diet. Chocolate, hard
cheeses or blue cheese (not quark or soft cheese) are frequent trigger factors and if so, should be avoided, as should
alcohol and tobacco.

Bidor 5%, 1 or 2 tablets three times daily, should be
taken regularly also between attacks. Take for about six
weeks, stop for four weeks, then take for another six weeks.
This treatment does not reduce the pain, but is a long-term
cure which increases the vitality of the nervous system.

Secale/Quartz, 10–15 pilules three times daily.

If an attack is threatening, take a small cup of strong
black coffee with lemon juice.

A homoeopathic medicine that has often proved useful
is Magnesium phosphoricum 6x or 12x.

Finding the right medicine is an art that calls for accu-
rate knowledge of the medicaments.

Hypoglycaema (low blood sugar levels) may sometimes also trigger a migraine. It is not sugar that is needed, however, but making sure the intervals between meals are not too long, eating a little every 3 to 5 hours.

Nervous conditions

Nervousness is essentially a problem arising from lifestyle. Tranquillizers of whatever kind only act for a time and do not get to the root of the trouble.

Nervous exhaustion

Kalium phosphoricum comp., 1 tablet three times daily; baths to which pine needle extract or Pine Bath Milk has been added; Wala Nerve Food.

Sleeplessness (insomnia), overexcitability

The possible causes of insomnia are so many that they cannot always be found. Often, however, quite minor things can stop us from getting to sleep — cold feet, for example. Alternating hot and cold footbaths at night may prove extremely helpful (see p.27). The body needs to be kept warm during sleep, and bedcovers should be adequate. Another cause may be a mattress that does not allow the body to get in the right position or allows cold to seep up from below. Another common obstacle to sleep is a succession of thoughts that 'keep going round and round in one's head' (the same individual will however sleep sweetly through a whole lecture). Sleep thus depends not only on physical but also mental aspects. Most people find it difficult to 'switch off' nowadays. In the old days, people were aware that on going to sleep they entered another world and they would prepare for this by saying their evening prayers. Something we can do today is to practise until we learn to govern the conscious mind to a point where the affairs of the day are left aside and other things, relating to art or religion, fill the mind (for soul hygiene, see Introduction).

Medicines that impose sleep should never be used for any length of time. More gentle remedies include: Weleda Sedative Tea — a cupful at night sweetened with honey; Avena sativa comp. or Avena sativa/Valeriana, 10 drops several times at night, as required; baths with Lavender Bath Milk added.

Weleda Calcium Supplement 2, ¼ teaspoonful at night. For children in particular, Bryophyllum Argento cultum 1%, 5–10 drops three times daily or just at night, is advisable, also warm body packs with mallow oil.

Herbal preparations with sedative and sleep-inducing actions are widely available. Most contain valerian and hops; other plants used are corydalis (Corydalis cava), passion flower (Passiflora coerulea) and oat (Avena sativa). They may be found at health food stores and some pharmacies and it may be necessary to try two or three before finding the one that suits individual needs.

These preparations do not enforce sleep but help to establish the natural process. They are not habit-forming. Their alterative properties are more important than any immediate effect and it often needs some weeks of regular use to achieve lasting results.

Night time sweating can also be an expression of over-excitability. With neurasthenia (fatigue, listlessness) sweatings can also occur during the day. For treatment see p.90.

Depression

As the name indicates, spirits are low in this condition. When induced by external circumstances or misfortunes, the term 'reactive' depression is used. 'Endogenous' depression describes a condition where no reason can be found for the mood change; it is much more difficult to deal with and may also take the form of manic-depressive disease, in which there are alternating phases of depression and excitement. This type of depression needs medical treatment, for it can lead to suicidal states.

Less acute depressions (such as latent depression) that nevertheless often make life, especially with others, extremely difficult are very common today. Stress and exhaustion can also lead to depression, especially during the second half of life, often causing total paralysis of inner life.

The individuals affected are tired and worn down, and at the same time unable to sleep; problems seem to pile up before them, with no way out. There is no point in trying to encourage them, and attempts at 'cheering them up' are liable to have the opposite effect, so that the sufferer withdraws even more, falls into despair and feels totally misunderstood.

In terms of human science based on spiritual research, this is not a 'nervous condition,' let alone 'neurological' or brain disease, but a metabolic disorder affecting primarily the liver. Particularly the milder or early stages respond well to medication that addresses the metabolism. The most important plant drug in this field is St John's wort (Hypericum). Preparations of this may be available from health food stores. A more lasting effect is achieved with Hypericum Auro cultum, 10 drops five times daily, particularly if taken in alternation with Hepar/Magnesium 4x, 10 drops three to five times daily. Injections of the latter have a more intensive effect. Problems of this kind clearly do

not come up out of the blue and therefore cannot be expected to go away instantly; treatment will therefore have
to continue for some weeks. A regular lifestyle should also
be established and there is need for the kind of soul hygiene described in the first chapter (see p.16).

Neuralgia, neuritis

Gently massage Aconitum comp., Oleum into the painful
areas or soak small pieces of material with the oil, place on
the painful areas and cover to keep warm. Leave in position
for several hours.

Take Arnica 20x, 8 drops twice daily, for some time, together with Apis 3x, 10 drops three times daily.

Dental care

It is now firmly established that sweet things cause dental
caries. Sticky products like chocolate, cakes, sweets and so
on, are worse than just sugar, for they tend to adhere more
to the teeth. It is therefore essential always to brush one's
teeth after eating anything sweet.

Toothpastes and mouthwashes with powerful disinfectant properties attack the oral flora and upset the natural
balance in the mucous membranes. For regular dental care
use Weleda Herbal Toothpaste or Weleda Salt Toothpaste
and Weleda Gargle and Mouthwash.

For bleeding gums, massage with undiluted Weleda Gargle and Mouthwash.

The teething of infants is made easier by giving
Chamomilla matricaria Rad. 3x, 5 drops three times daily,
possibly in alternation with Kieserite 4x.

Gingivitis, stomatitis, dental abscess

Rinse with Calendula Lotion, 1 teaspoonful to a glass of warm water, retaining the liquid in the mouth or using it as a rinse. See also under Sore mouth on p.59.

Periodontosis (receding gums)

This is not a local disease but a condition affecting the whole organism. The basis for improvement is a good quality diet (see p.22f).

Apart from dental treatment, apply Ceratum Ratanhia comp. several times daily, especially after brushing the teeth at night, to the mucous membrane and/or gums, which should be as dry as possible.

Sensitive teeth

Take Kieserite 6x, 8–10 drops three times daily; after about a month, Kieserite 20x, 10 drops twice daily.

Toothache

After dental treatment or before a visit to the dentist is possible: take Allium cepa 3x, 10 drops at hourly intervals, alternating with Mercurius vivus naturalis 6x, 1 tablet. After dental surgery or extractions: take Arnica 3x, 5–7 drops initially at hourly intervals and after some days 10 drops three times a day.

Ear, nose and throat diseases

Earache (otitis)

In children this is often due to a middle ear infection. First aid measures consist in keeping warm and applying dry camomile bags or, better, onion poultices.

Levisticum Radix 3x, 7 drops to be taken in water every hour or half hour. This may be alternated with Silicea comp. Locally apply Levisticum 10% oil; put 10–20 drops on a teaspoon and warm gently over a flame, take up in some cotton wool and introduce this slowly into the ear as hot as it can be borne. Cover the ear with a woollen cloth.

Nosebleed (epistaxis)

This is quite common and usually harmless. A doctor should be consulted if nosebleeds occur more frequently.

During a nosebleed, do not lie down but sit up. Do not blow your nose. People who are liable to nosebleeds should keep at hand a supply of Stibium met. prep. 6x powder, and take a pinch of this like snuff as required.

Sinusitis

Not every blocked nose is 'sinusitis.' Chronic catarrh has become increasingly more common in recent years, especially with children. The reasons for this vary, but it is often a problem of not being warm enough. With chronic conditions or at the beginning of an acute inflammation (not when the very acute stage has been reached) inhalation treatments can make an enormous difference. Bend the head over a bowl of steaming camomile tea and drape a bath towel over head and bowl; inhale the vapours, which should be as hot as possible, through the nose. When the water temperature has gone down a little, add one or two drops of a volatile oil such as eucalyptus, pumilio or dwarf pine, Olbas or Japanese Peppermint. Go to bed afterwards, keeping the head well covered to keep the warmth in. An even better method is to generate one's own heat by physical exertion. In either case it is important to take care that one does not get cold or chilled afterwards.

The lack of warmth may also originate in the abdomen or the legs. It is therefore most important to get warm and keep warm. Mustard footbaths have also proved effective (a handful of mustard powder to a bucket of warm water; immerse legs for ten minutes to just below the knee).

Horseradish is an outstanding remedy for all types of sinusitis; it may be taken internally and applied in poultices (see *Home Nursing* section under *Further Reading*), with freshly grated horseradish put on a small piece of cloth and applied to the forehead or cheeks. The resulting skin irritation will among other things restore secretory function. Take great care not to let the horseradish come in contact with the eyes, covering the eye area with Vaseline ointment if necessary.

In many cases, dietary imbalance is the underlying cause, mainly excess of protein, which is so common today. With children in particular it will sometimes only be possible to get results if protein intake is limited for some weeks and care taken to see that they do not have sugar, sweets or refined flour products (including soft drinks).

Medication will often only prove effective if attention is

given to the above. Silicea comp. (5–10 pilules at hourly intervals) is recommended, as are the use of spa salts (see below), and camomile tea.

Nasal catarrh (coryza)

Nasal catarrh is a nuisance but not a disease in its own right. Suppression with decongestants is not advisable, as it may in some cases cause the problem to shift further down and result in bronchitis or a chronic catarrhal state depending on the decongestant used. In the acute stage, a few drops of Japanese Peppermint Oil, Olbas Oil or a similar volatile oil put on a handkerchief and inhaled give rapid relief. The same oils may also be taken by mouth (1–2 drops on a little sugar). A highly effective method is to draw up luke-warm salt water through the nose or introduce a small roll of cotton wool soaked in salt water into the nose.

For a supportive measure, take hot footbaths with rising water temperature to which a teaspoonful of Rosemary Bath Milk or the juice of half a lemon has been added. Care should always be taken to see that the feet are warm and the body is kept warm (for more details, see *Further Reading*).

For a running nose, take Arsenicum album 10x, 5 drops at hourly intervals, possibly in alternation with Allium cepa 3x. Locally, Nose Balm may be applied; Nose Balm Mild for children.

For chronic coryza, see under frontal sinusitis.

Regular application of Catarrh Cream 2 is advisable if nasal catarrhs are frequent. Spa salts such as Vichy, Carlsbad or Ems Salt have proved effective as a gargle or for rinsing the nose; use about a teaspoonful to ¼ litre (quart) of warm water. An ointment made with genuine Ems Salt is helpful with both acute and chronic catarrh.

A dry nose or throat may be responsible for acute catarrh developing. Again the regular use of the above-mentioned ointments or balms will prove helpful. Damaged mucous membranes of the nose may be helped to regenerate by Coldastop, an oil containing vitamin A and E, which should be used regularly for a time. Oleum Rhinale I and II have been found to be particularly effective with dry nasal mucous. Soledum nasal drops contain an extract of chamomile that reduces inflammation.

Hay fever

Hay fever is not a cold; it is caused by the pollen from grasses and/or flowers and affects individuals who are sensitive to such pollen. The condition therefore occurs only during the season when the plants produce pollen. Hypersensitivity is frequently part of a generalized 'allergic reaction' and calls for general treatment; local applications merely suppress the symptoms. A general alterative effect is achieved by reducing protein and salt intake to an absolute minimum during acute attacks. It may sometimes even be necessary to cut out protein altogether and take an almost salt-free diet. It is also advisable to drink as little as possible at this time. Bowel function needs attention, and even if the individual does not suffer from constipation the bowel flora, on which our health depends to a great extent, may be far from normal. Alterative measures such as eating sauerkraut may be necessary, or eating nothing but cooked carrots or raw apples for a few days.

Relief may be gained by diluting Gencydo liquid with water to which a little salt has been added and drawing this up through the nose. Gencydo may also be given by injection to achieve the necessary alterative effect; it should be given before the hay fever season starts, that is, from about

February onwards. An even better method is to use one ampoule of Gencydo daily with an inhaler or aerosol spray. Internally, a homeopathic hay fever preparation such as Nelson's Hay Fever Tablets may be taken, again starting around February.

It is possible to suppress hay fever symptoms rapidly by using powerful drugs such as cortisone. From the biological point of view this is not a good method, as the drug intervenes in the hormone metabolism and reduces the ability to produce inflammatory reactions. This may have serious consequences for the whole constitution.

Acute sore throat (tonsillitis)

Cinnabar (Merc. sulph.) 6x, 1 tablet at hourly intervals. Gargle with Bolus Eucalypti comp., 1 teaspoonful of the powder in half a glass of warm water. Drink sage tea and also use this to rinse the mouth. For local use: Echinacea Mouth Spray.

Peritonsillar abscess (quinsy)

This requires medical treatment and supervision. As a first-aid measure, take Mercurius cyanatus 4x (7 drops at hourly intervals). Constipation is common with this condition and should be treated with a laxative tea or an enema. Equisetum (horsetail) tea or Equisetum 4x may be taken to help elimination of toxins via the kidneys. Apply a lemon compress. Drink sage tea and also use it as a gargle. For further details, see works cited under *Home Nursing* in *Further Reading*.

Chronic tonsilitis, susceptibility to sore throats

Cinnabar (Merc. sulph.) 6x, 1 tablet twice daily for about
8–10 weeks; 2–4 week interval, then repeat. Drink sage tea
regularly for some time.

Sore mouth (stomatitis), mouth ulcers

These are often, but not always, due to unbalanced diet. A
short period on raw food or a low- or no-protein diet may
have an alterative effect. Local treatment consists in rinsing
with dilute Calendula Essence (1 tablespoonful to ¼ litre,
¼ quart of water) and then applying Bolus Eucalypti comp.
powder to the affected areas, leaving it to act for as long as
possible.

Weleda Mouthwash has good disinfectant properties as
it is based on essential oils.

Thuja occidentalis 4x, 8 drops three times daily, may be
taken for four weeks. The juice of a lemon with meals, or
diluted and drunk during the day, supports the above measures.

Bad breath

This may be due to a variety of causes, among them mouth
ulcers, poor dental hygiene, infected tonsils, gastrointestinal disorders, liver disease, or even hunger.

Chlorophyll preparations such as Clorets have a general
deodorant effect that deals with the symptom but not the
underlying cause.

Hoarseness

Anise/Pyrites 3x, 1 tablet at hourly intervals. Externally, apply massage oil to the throat. Iceland moss is a popular herbal remedy available as pastilles and other preparations.

Respiratory diseases

Cough, bronchitis

General measures include producing a sweat, inhalation of essential oils such as eucalyptus oil, Oleum Pini sylvest., or mixtures such as Olbas Oil or Japanese Peppermint Oil (for instance, Obbekjaer's), Sanavita Baokang Oil, Chinese Oil and others. The latter are steam-distilled, partly dementholised mint oil, which is also used as an ingredient in many other volatile oils. They do not affect the action of other medicines, including potentised preparations. Warnings issued that these oils make homoeopathic medicines ineffective are due to a misunderstanding. Put a few drops on a handkerchief or pillow or in boiling water, so that they evaporate. These oils give great relief.

A number of useful products such as Vick's Vapour Rub are available for chest rubs. Good teas are Sytra Tea and good quality herb teas for coughs and bronchitis. Drink a cup of the infusion (do not boil) three to six times daily, adding woodland honey if desired. For irritating coughs, use Weleda Cough Drops, 10 drops once an hour in some warm water or on sugar; this relieves the irritation but does not suppress the cough. A few drops of camphor oil applied

externally around the throat also help to relieve the irritation. Anise/Pyrites 3x, 1 tablet every one or two hours, is
particularly useful for hoarseness and for bronchitis when
it is high up in the chest. A mixture of the following homeopathic potencies — Ipecacuanha 5x, Drosera 3x and
Cuprum aceticum 4x — or similar may be taken as cough
drops. Herbal expectorants are also available; they contain
Plantago (ribwort plantain), Tussilago (coltsfoot) or Thy-
mus (thyme); for instance, Potter's Balm of Gilead Cough
Mixture. Weleda expectorants are Lichenes comp. and
Cough Elixir. Pure Thyme Oil is sold under a number of
different names. It is also contained in compound preparations such as Angocin, Tixylix.

Chronic bronchitis

A doctor needs to be consulted to establish the cause;
heavy smokers, for instance, tend to suffer from chronic
bronchitis. Alterative measures include regular sweat baths
(once or twice a week) to which essential oils have been
added (Oleum Pini sylvest. extract or products containing
pumilio or dwarf pine oil are particularly useful) and mustard compresses applied to the back. Resistance is improved by taking products based on Equisetum (horsetail)
juice.

Acute and chronic conditions of the lung may respond
to herbal antibiotics. It has been shown that the aromatic
principles contained in onions and other highly odorous
plants have a powerful effect in preventing bacteria from
multiplying, more powerful than antibiotics such as
penicillin and others that are obtained from moulds.
Nasturtium, horseradish and other plants have similar
properties.

Angocin is an example. It may be taken to treat all inflammatory conditions in the throat and lung region and also urinary infections. The pack gives exact details of how to use it.

Extracts from medical plants that are lung-specific have been mentioned above.

Whooping cough

Whooping cough is a troublesome childhood illness that is not dangerous unless there are complications. The latter are generally avoided by refraining from the wrong kind of treatment, that is, medicines that bring down a fever and suppress the cough.

The key to management is calmness and common sense, and a light diet containing no milk or milk products. High altitudes (above 1000 m, 3000 ft) give rapid relief.

Anthroposophical medicines include Pertudoron 1 and 2 given hourly in alternation, 2–8 drops, depending on age.

Products based on ivy leaf extracts give rapid relief. Examples are Hederka and Prospan.

Asthma

There are different types of asthma, ranging from purely psychosomatic to what is known as 'allergic' asthma. The latter is caused by inhaling substances to which the patient is sensitive. Once a particular sensitivity has been diagnosed the substance in question should be avoided, but this is not always possible. A period in the mountains or at the seaside will usually be beneficial, but individual needs differ. Asthma is a serious illness and medical advice should always be sought.

Below, some general alterative measures are suggested.

They are intended to give more than temporary relief on a long-term basis. Other medicines may be needed in acute attacks, and these are not designed for continuous use. The medicines listed below are used to stimulate the organism so that it becomes able to overcome the disease, that is, to initiate a cure, and that means long-term use. Take 10–20 drops of Quercus 1x (10%) in the mornings and 10–20 drops of Veronica officinalis 2x at night. Alternatively, Petasites comp. cum Quercu (10 pilules) in the mornings and Petasites comp. cum Veronica (10 pilules) at night. Cuprum aceticum 4x (5–10 drops at about 4 and 6 p.m.) is a basic remedy specially indicated when there is aggravation at night, which is common with asthmatics.

Pneumonium LA is a well proven herbal preparation of fresh Petasites (butterbur) (20–30 drops three times daily). Good quality asthma teas (Kneipp) are also helpful.

With children, a short period on an alkaline diet (as far as possible avoiding meat, fish, eggs and dairy products and all but wholemeal grain products) is often beneficial.

Heart, circulation and blood

Heart conditions

Medical advice should always be sought.

A weak heart in elderly persons has been found to respond well to preparations of hawthorn (Crataegus), for instance, Crataegus Drops and Tablets.

For sudden sharp pains in the heart when there is no organic cause, take Spigelia anthelmia 4x, 7 drops three times daily.

A general 'heart tonic' made with homeopathic potencies often proves useful with a 'nervous heart,' that is, the functional heart symptoms that may develop after over-work or illness.

Cardiodoron A is a basic medicine that maintains a healthy functional balance in the cardiovascular system, preventing more serious heart complaints. Take 15 drops three times daily before meals.

Cardiac weakness may be treated with mixtures containing menthol, camphor, Crataegus (hawthorn), valerian or Convallaria (lily-of-the-valley) that are best prescribed by a doctor.

Angina needs medical care and supervision. Arm baths of the kind described in the section on water treatments (see p.26f) have proved helpful as a supportive measure. A basic medicament is Crataegus (see above), and also Magnesium phos. 3x, 1 tablet (or pinch of powder) three times daily over an extended period.

A number of organic magnesium compounds are available, all of them relieve the spasms.

Circulatory disorders

Both low and high blood pressure can cause unpleasant and also dangerous general problems.

With **low blood pressure** (hypotension), add a few drops of Rosemary Bath Milk to the washwater or put them on the face flannel in the mornings; add more salt to your food; plenty of physical exercise in careful dosage, that is, slowly increasing the amount done; take a preparation of whole extract of Sarothamnus scoparius (broom), 20 drops three times daily. Symptoms experienced with hypotension, for instance, tiredness or a tendency to faint, are generally harmless. People with low blood pressure generally live longer than those with high blood pressure.

Many people suffer from **high blood pressure** (hypertension) without even being aware of it, and indeed may feel active and full of energy because of it. That is only to begin with, however; later — sometimes only years later — dangerous consequences develop, among them congestion in the head, cirrhosis of the kidney, sleeplessness and strokes. The best prevention is to have your blood pressure checked regularly and make the necessary changes in lifestyle sooner rather than later. These include a low-salt diet, reduced protein intake (a vegetarian diet would be best), light but regular physical activity, general mental hygiene, that is, learning to 'switch off.' See that there are periods of rest when you do something else than what normally fills the day (see p.15f). Older people may find it extremely helpful to take garlic, for instance, Cardiomax Garlic Perles. Medicines based on mistletoe and hawthorn may be indicated (Gerard's range of herbal products includes a Hawthorn preparation, for instance). Please note that mistletoe tea should be used, not mistletoe extract.

Fainting

Some people, especially young people and particularly young women, may faint after standing for some time, if the air is bad or from powerful emotions. This is usually only a temporary syncope or circulatory collapse. Fresh air and the application of cologne to the forehead will almost always bring the person round. Even better are Rosemary Bath Milk or Melissa comp. put on the palms of the hand and inhaled. People who are unconscious should never be given anything to drink, as this may cause them to choke. When recovered, give repeated doses of Cardiodoron A, which also serves to prevent further attacks.

Varicose veins

These develop when the veins that take the blood from the periphery to the heart are abnormally dilated. On the one hand this is a cardiovascular problem, on the other it involves connective tissue weakness. Support hose or elastic bandages can help to prevent the condition from getting worse.

A number of excellent herbal products are available for both internal use and external application; they are generally based on horse chestnut (Aesculus) extracts and wych-hazel (Hamamelis) and address both causes.

Weleda Skin Tone Lotion has proved helpful as an external application. A herbal product for tired legs is Phyto-varix Massage Gel.

Individual veins often become inflamed (phlebitis) and in that case a doctor should be consulted. Having done so, the following may prove helpful: wear elastic bandages; when resting, apply compresses with Borago 20% lotion, a teaspoonful to ¼ litre (quart) of lukewarm water.

Leg cramps are common with circulatory disorders of the legs and during pregnancy. In addition to the herbal medicines used for varicose veins, a homeopathic preparation, Cuprum arsen. (olivenite) 6x is helpful, a pinch of powder three times daily. The same preparation is even more effective if given by injection, but this requires medical supervision.

Magnesium preparations are also indicated (see p.64).

Anaemia

Anaemia is a symptom of disease, not a disease in itself. The causes have to be found and treated, and a doctor should therefore be consulted.

Being pale does not necessarily mean being anaemic. This applies also in the case of children who may look 'anaemic' for quite different reasons.

Anaemia is frequently, but not always, due to iron deficiency, which means, of course, that iron has to be given. Excessive blood loss may cause iron deficiency anaemia, for example. Many different iron preparations are available and may be taken in this case. They are almost always organic iron compounds, some with added vitamins or other substances.

It may happen, however, that iron preparations prove ineffective or are effective only for a limited period. This may indicate an inability to take up sufficient iron, metabolize it properly, or retain it. In this case it is useless to give iron preparations. Instead, the body's ability to deal with iron needs to be stimulated, which may be done by giving spinach, for instance. A common objection to this is that spinach does not contain enough iron and therefore will be useless in treating iron deficiency anaemia. It is true that spinach contains relatively little iron, but that is not the point. Eating spinach encourages the organism to take up iron and metabolize it. A particularly effective method is to add one third of fresh stinging nettle leaves to the spinach. They will not affect the taste much but give excellent support to iron metabolism. Nettle leaf tea taken regularly, especially in spring, has a similar effect; the taste can be improved by adding peppermint and lemon balm leaves.

When haemoglobin levels are tested to establish whether an individual is anaemic or not, it must be remembered that some individuals normally have lower levels that are perfectly adequate. This applies particularly to women. The difference in iron levels compared to those of men are not due to the blood lost through menstrual discharge and cannot be changed by giving iron. It is rather a characteristic of the whole female organization that tends to be particularly common in women with blond or reddish blond hair.

Before puberty children also have relatively lower iron levels than adults. Iron deficiency may show itself in their case in failure to thrive, lack of appetite, lack of drive, and so on. A stinging nettle preparation grown in soil treated with potentized iron, Ferrum per Urtica 1%, will be found useful, 5–10 drops (depending on the age of the child) three times daily. After about four weeks, change to Anaemodoron/Gentian, 10–12 drops three times daily. Again it is not the iron as such that matters, but stimulating the organism to utilize iron. Nutrition is obviously important, too. Wholemeal bread is rich in minerals and iron, white bread on the other hand does not contain adequate amounts of these.

Acids help iron uptake, and anaemic people often have a longing for lemon or vinegar.

Swollen glands

Unless due to an acute condition, swollen glands are a constitutional problem. The tonsils and adenoids are most commonly affected, breathing is more difficult, so that children keep their mouths open and are constantly suffering from catarrh. This is also known as a lymphatic constitution.

A stay at the seaside is often beneficial. Homeopathic preparations such as Barium iodatum 4x or Juglans regia 1x (10 drops three times daily) help the organism to deal with this kind of constitution. Another useful remedy is Juglans regia comp. (Wala).

Archangelica comp. ointment may be applied locally. Berberis ointment (Berberis, fructus, 10%) applied over the bladder for two or three months, acts from the opposite pole.

Digestion and nutrition

Acute stomach upset (gastritis)

Fasting is indicated. Keep the abdomen warm, apply a hot body compress (see *Home Nursing* under *Further Reading*). Take camomile tea, possibly with a small amount of wormwood added. Oat gruel made with water should be the first food taken after fasting.

Bitters are particularly helpful, for instance, Gentiana lutea 5%, repeated doses of 10 drops each.

In cases of **nausea** or **vomiting:** Nux vomica 4x, 5 drops put on the tongue every thirty minutes. Ipecacuanha 6x, may be alternated with Nux vomica.

Sensation of **bloated stomach** or feeling of fullness after heavy, indigestible food: Artemisia comp., several doses of 10 drops each, preferably in hot water.

For **'acidity'** eructations, apply pressure over the stomach: Amara Drops, 7–10 drops several times daily.

For **heartburn:** Robinia comp., in the acute stage 10 pilules every fifteen minutes. For chronic heartburn, 10 pilules three times daily before meals.

Chronic gastric complaints and indigestion

A doctor should be consulted. Bad breath may be a sign of gastroenterites (see p.71).

An 'irritable or nervous stomach' can be treated by drinking centaury (Centaurium) or wormwood (Artemisia abs.) tea; a useful mixture is Pinella Tea, a cupful twice a day, or, better, drink that amount sip by sip throughout the day. Amara Drops, 5–7 drops several times a day.

Indigestion, dyspepsia, lack of appetite

The right kind of seasoning, using herbs and spices, may give relief, something we often know instinctively. First to be considered are hot spices such as paprika, curry and chili pepper (not black pepper). These, and our native herbs such as lovage, tarragon, basil, thyme and many others, help the digestion, even if liver function is on the weak side. Bitters, particularly if taken as an aperitif before meals, stimulate gastric secretion. Piquant seasonings, mixed pickles, for instance, and mustard, specially help the digestion of proteins.

Salt has absolutely nothing to do with digestion. It does not aid digestion or increase the appetite, but it does add savour. Sadly, 'season well' is usually taken to mean 'add lots of salt.' A good cook manages with relatively little salt. If salt intake has to be reduced, for instance, with high blood pressure or kidney disease, salt can be almost completely replaced by the above herbs and spices.

For chronic complaints, take Digestodoron or Amara Drops, 20 drops three times daily before meals, for three months. Also, for a rapid action in acute cases: Gentiana lutea 5%, Artemisia comp. (see above).

Gastroenteritis, diarrhoea

Diarrhoea and vomiting and loss of appetite serve to clean out the gastrointestinal canal, so that initially at least they have a positive purpose. The first food taken after this is grated raw apple (with nothing added) or cooked carrots. It is important to apply heat to the abdomen, preferably in form of a body compress or otherwise with a hot water bottle (see works cited for *Home Nursing* under *Further Reading*).

The following charcoal preparations help to remove toxins, particularly with summer diarrhoeas, and may be safely taken in any amount: Carbo Betulae comp., 3–4 tablets, Carbo coffeae.

A purely herbal product of camomile and tormentil may also be used. If there is also cardiovascular weakness (cold sweats), take Veratrum album 4x, 5 drops every hour. These preparations are intended for use in the acute stage only.

Diarrhoea in infants can be life-threatening because fluid levels go down very quickly. Always give unsweetened tea (camomile or possibly also weak ordinary tea) instead of the usual bottle feed. Sugar and honey should not be used as they increase fermentation in the gut and therefore aggravate the diarrhoea. A doctor must always be consulted if infants are losing weight rapidly.

Measures to prevent gastroenteritis when travelling are discussed on p.38.

Hepatitis

See p.39

Flatulence (wind)

Flatulence usually indicates either a weak digestion or something wrong with the diet. It is obviously a good idea to avoid indigestible foods as much as possible. Experience has shown that these are usually members of the cabbage family and pulses, especially beans. The type of fertilizer used plays a major role in the digestibility of these vegetables, and this is easily demonstrated in the case of cabbage. Biodynamically grown cabbage is much better tolerated by sensitive people than cabbage grown on land fertilized with liquid farmyard manure or chemical fertilizers. It has also been known for centuries that cabbage is much more digestible if made into sauerkraut. Another way of making cabbage more digestible is to add caraway to it. Caraway, anise, coriander and other herbs and spices added to the dough also make bread more digestible. 'Intolerance' is frequently merely due to the wrong foods being combined. Many foods (wholemeal bread, for example) may cause fermentation and irritation merely because they have been combined with sugar products. The same applies to sweetened desserts.

Infants are helped by massaging the tummy with calamus oil or fennel oil.

A weak digestion can be corrected by using the measures given in the section on indigestion above.

Carminative mixtures containing caraway oil, fennel oil, tincture of calamus, belladonna and valerian, 10 drops three times daily before meals, are useful, or Carbo Betulae 5%/Ol. aeth. Carvi 1%, 2 tablets three times a day before meals or more frequent doses.

Constipation

This is one of the commonest problems in our present age. The causes are many, above all changes in diet. Many modern foods are highly refined and contain little of the roughage or fibre needed to stimulate bowel activity. White flour is produced by removing the bran that wholemeal products still contain. Bran can be added to foods; it absorbs a large volume of liquid and acts as a bulking agent, so that there is usually no need to take anything else for constipation. It is obviously better not to remove the bran from the grain in the first place, and wholegrain products are always preferable.

Sedentary lifestyles and lack of physical exercise are a further cause. Apart from this, constipation is partly due to constitutional factors, and in spite of refined foods and sedentary habits not everyone suffers from constipation.

The condition will often be no more than a nuisance to those who suffer from it, but inadequate elimination can also be a sign of poor metabolic activity. In the course of time this may be an aggravating factor in chronic diseases, preventing a cure. The bowel then produces toxins rather than removing them. Almost all cancer patients are found to have been constipated for years, for instance, and whilst it is not possible to cure cancer by dealing with the problem of constipation, improving metabolic function will almost always have a favourable effect on chronic diseases.

Laxatives should be reserved for acute situations; they should not be used for longer periods. The fact that they give rapid and reliable results means that people tend to use them freely, not realizing that they are habit-forming and that their bowels become even less active than before. Years of laxative abuse can cause serious damage to health, mainly changes in mineral metabolism that may be so profound that they are extremely difficult to correct.

Caution is also indicated with laxatives during pregnancy, for they may cause abortion.

If there is need to empty the bowel immediately, which is the case, for instance, with all febrile diseases, purulent sore throats and also many chronic diseases, the safest and quickest method is an enema, using water or camomile tea at body temperature.

Rapid results may be achieved with suppositories that produce carbon dioxide in the bowel, and these can also be safely used with children. A glycerine enema softens stools and stimulates bowel movement; glycerine suppositories and ready-made enemas are available.

Where diet is concerned, linseed is the first to consider. It acts both as a bulking agent and a lubricant. Whole seeds may be soaked for twelve hours in water and 1–2 tablespoons of this taken, or they may be freshly crushed and added to muesli. Commercial linseed preparations are also available. Ortisan and Dual-lax are useful products. A good method is to cook whole rye or wheat grain like rice and serve with vegetables, though this may cause flatulence in some people who are susceptible.

Raw sauerkraut acts as an alterative on the bowel. One half to one teaspoonful of mustard seeds, taken whole, also stimulate bowel action. Another well-tried method is to soak prunes for twelve hours in lukewarm water and then eat the fruit and drink the water. Dried figs may also be eaten.

Lactose encourages the fermentative activity of intestinal bacteria. It is only slightly sweet and can be added to foods. A similar substance, lactulose, is available, but consult your doctor before using it.

Medicinal springs and their salts have been used through the centuries. Epsom salts are an example. They stimulate the production of bile and also reduce the absorption of water from the gut so that stools remain soft. Such salts are suitable for a limited course of treatment but not for long-term use. Dissolve a teaspoonful in warm water and take in small sips on an empty stomach in the mornings; the dose may need to be adjusted to individual requirements. A bowel movement will follow one or two hours later.

A number of plants or parts of plants also have instant laxative actions, among them figs, prunes, cascara and tamarind; preparations of aloes or senna leaves are even more powerful, and there are many of these on the market. They are largely herbal and therefore may be called 'natural,' but caution is indicated with long-term use and also during pregnancy (see above). Some of the many products are Arcolax (a psyllium preparation), rhubarb mixtures or compound rhubarb tablets, Laxadoron, senna syrup (based on senna leaf) and Senokot (based on senna fruit). Clairo Tea is taken at night (infused, not boiled).

Most important of all is getting the bowels to become active of their own accord again. This calls on the one hand for physical activity and exercise and on the other for meals to be taken in a proper rhythm and to contain plenty of fibre. Bowel action is also stimulated by massaging copper ointment (Cuprum met. prep. 0.4%) into the abdomen using a clockwise circular motion.

The question as to whether someone is suffering from constipation or not has to do not with the frequency or regularity of bowel movements but with the consistency of the stools. Rock-hard stools are just as pathological as regular stools that show a high degree of putrefaction (smelly and much gas).

Worms

The most common worm infestations in Central and Northern Europe are:
1 **Tapeworms**: these require supervised medical treatment. They are usually passed on through raw meat.
2 **Roundworms** (about 10 cm long): a safe preparation is a product containing papain and specific activators (Vermizym), given as directed, taking account of age. Roundworm eggs are mainly passed on through the practice of sewage top dressing to fertilize the soil, which is still used in some areas.
3 **Threadworms** (pinworms): these are very thin and 1–2 mm long; almost all children have them at some time or other. They are harmless but can be troublesome if present in large numbers and because they cause anal irritation. The simplest cure is giving practically nothing but carrots for several days. Garlic is also effective, either added to food on a regular basis or used intensively for a short period. Herrings (not other fish) can also be used for this purpose.

Hygiene is most important, with the whole anal region carefully washed after stools and above all at bedtime. The intestinal environment is improved by giving a tansy preparation such as Tanacetum Strath. Strath, 20 drops three times daily, or Cina comp.m 5 – 10 drops three times daily. These preparations have to be taken regularly for some time (6 – 10 weeks), however. They change the intestinal environment and do not kill worms directly.

Haemorrhoids (piles)

It is important to ensure that stools are soft.

Weleda Stibium comp. suppositories or herbal suppositories containing wych-hazel (Hamamelis) and horse
chestnut (Aesculus) may be used once or twice a day, after
stools.

Hamamelis ointment and Aesculus ointment may also
be used externally, and, particularly in the acute stage, an
ointment or suppositories containing an extract of
butcher's broom (Ruscus aculeatus).

Liver and gall-bladder conditions

Diet plays a vital role in this, whatever may sometimes be
said to the contrary. Serious liver or gall-bladder disease always requires medical treatment. There are however many
chronic conditions where the following measures may be
used in support of medical treatment.

Liver

A special diet should be taken only to begin with — light
rye or wholemeal bread, total fats not to exceed 60g (2 oz)
per day, depending on the severity of the condition. Eat
less fat rather than more. No fried foods, coffee or sugar.
Milk is best in form of sour milk or yoghurt. Quark (low-
fat soft white cheese) may be taken in any amount. Eat little per meal, but five meals a day. Later the diet need be
less strict and should consist mainly of fresh vegetables
and fruit, nothing tinned, bottled or frozen. Pickled cucum-
bers — lactic fermented, not in vinegar — are specially

recommended, as are other lactic fermented vegetables, sauerkraut and sour milk.

During the acute stage, complete bedrest is mandatory, with warm compresses applied over the liver at least once a day, preferably yarrow (Achillea mil.) compresses.

The best tolerated and most universal fat is butter or cream, both to be used with discretion as part of the total fat allowance. Some people do however find that they tolerate oil better; individuals differ in this respect. As far as possible avoid heating fats. The more and longer they are heated, the less digestible and indeed harmful do they become. Patients should therefore avoid all fried and deep-fried foods. A basic medication is Hepatodoron, 1 or 2 tablets three times daily before meals or 3 or 4 tablets at night, for quite a long time.

Carduus marianus 1x, 10–20 drops three times daily before meals, has proved most useful and rapid in action. Young dandelion leaves, as a salad or as juice (health food stores) are recommended, and Hepar/Stannum 4x, 10 drops three times daily before meals.

Gall-bladder

Avoid stone fruits; caution is indicated with oil, fried and roasted foods. Take Choleodoron, 10 drops three times daily after meals, for a relatively long time, in the acute stage 10 drops in hot water every twenty minutes. Oxalis comp., 10 drops three times daily before meals, alternating with Magnesium phosphoricum 6x dil. If biliary colic threatens, take 8–10 drops of these every thirty minutes.

Kidney and bladder conditions

Chronic kidney diseases are very serious conditions; a doctor should always be consulted.

Kidney diseases are often diagnosed too late. It is essential, therefore, to have the urine tested after any purulent sore throat or other throat disease. If nephritis does develop afterwards, bedrest, warmth and dietary restrictions are absolutely essential. The strain can be taken off the kidney by keeping fluid intake to a minimum for a limited period; the diet should be salt-free and very low in protein. Failure to allow full recovery from acute nephritis, even in a mild case, will result in chronic nephritis, which is difficult to treat and frequently proves fatal.

Chronic nephritis

Consult a doctor. In general terms, eat a low-salt diet; keep warm, avoid getting chilled; avoid physical exertion, as in sports.

Equisetum tea, a cupful two or three times daily. Boil in a covered pan for 15–20 minutes; merely infusing it is not enough. Make peppermint tea or lemon balm tea with the resulting decoction to improve the flavour.

Renodoron, 1 tablet three times daily, for at least three months, two or three weeks break, then repeat. Equisetum cum Sulphure tostum 3x, trit., a pinch of powder three times daily, in addition to Renodoron or alternating with it week by week. Apply Cuprum met.0.4% ointment to kidney region at night. Wear something warm over the kidneys. Food Combining (the Hay diet) has proved effective.

Pyelitis

'Urinary tract infection' is a common condition nowadays. It is usually treated with antibiotics, which give rapid results but do not cure the condition, so that there will soon be a recurrence. The underlying cause is a weakness in the kidney system and a disorder of heat metabolism. Both need to be addressed for long-term results, using measures such as the following:

Take plenty of fluids, hot sitz baths (not full baths), take care that the feet are warm. Regularly take Equisetum tea (see above), Weleda Kidney Tea or one of the herbal kidney and bladder teas that are generally available.

Lachesis 12x, 8 drops three times daily. Thuja Argento culta 0.1%, 8 drops three times daily. Take one of these for two weeks, then the other, continuing like this for a long period.

The bacteria found to be responsible for the condition in the majority of cases often respond well to a diet that alternates between acid and alkaline foods, so that the urine alternates between being acid and alkaline for five days at a time. This is done by taking half a gramme of vitamin C three times daily and drinking bearberry tea during the acid phase; during the alkaline phase, meat, cola drinks and anything that makes the urine sour should be avoided. Another method is to take a good pinch of sodium bicarbonate three times daily. Many people will find it easier to alternate every seven days. The method can be extremely helpful, particularly with chronic conditions. The disease is liable to cause severe kidney damage, and it is always advisable to consult a doctor.

Cystitis

Application of heat as above.

Cantharis comp., 10–15 pilules four or five times daily. Apply Argentum 0.4% ointment to the region over the bladder daily.

Take bearberry or a herbal bladder tea.

Weak, irritable or nervous bladder

If no organic cause is found, herbal bladder medicines containing Sabal serrulata (saw palmetto) and/or Echinacea may prove helpful. Pumpkin seeds and preparations made from these are also beneficial.

Bedwetting (enuresis)

The cause should be established — children may be going back to an earlier phase of development because a little brother or sister has arrived and they feel they need more attention; contrariness; sleep too deep; undiagnosed bladder or kidney disease such as urinary tract infection, and so on. In most cases, the mental and psychological situation needs to be considered in support of medical treatment.

The latter will depend on the individual situation. A useful herbal product containing pumpkin seed oil and extracts of kava, sweet sumach and hops is Fink Cysto Capsules; treatment will have to be given for some time and the best method is to start with relatively high doses and gradually reduce these. Similar products may be available.

Prostate problems

Symptoms may be relatively minor to begin with, but a doctor should always be consulted, as they may be early signs of a more serious condition.

Avoid irritants in the diet — no pepper, little milk, no milk products at night and drink as little at possible at night.

A wide range of well-proven herbal and homeopathic medicines are available that often prove highly effective particularly in the early stages. Look for products containing Agropyron repens (couch grass), Cucurbita pepo (pumpkin seed oil or flour), Echinacea (rudbeckia), Populus tremula (aspen), Sabal serrulata (saw palmetto), Solidago virgaurea (goldenrod), Urtica dioica (stinging nettle). Medication needs to be long-term (about three months).

A simple trick helps the awkward problem of having to get out of bed to go the toilet during the night. Eat something salty — a piece of salt herring, pickled cucumber or the like — and drink little before going to bed. Avoid salt in the mornings and drink plenty — half a litre (½ quart) of herb tea, for example — to get rid of the salt and water accumulated overnight. The effect is even greater if ordinary tea is taken as well in the mornings; this is usually better tolerated than coffee which may prove an irritant.

Muscles, bones and joints

Sciatica

General measures: keep warm, induce sweats, apply local heat with hot compresses using either diluted (1:10) Arnica Essence, or ointment containing lyophilized bee venom, or ABC liniment (Aconite, Belladonna and Chloroform). Apply to the painful area.

Rheumatic conditions

These include a wide variety of diseases, all of them involving sharp pain, joint and muscle inflammation and limitation of movement. In the industrialized world about one in three people suffer from some form of rheumatic condition. This type of disease has thus become a social issue, as expensive treatments will often be needed for a period of many years and sufferers may be forced to take early retirement.

More than one hundred different diseases fall under this general heading, some of them fully researched. It is known, for example, that there is a hereditary element with some of them and that with others the wrong kind of physical stress may be a trigger or aggravating factor. Unbalanced diet also plays a significant, though frequently disregarded, role. Previous infections, hypersensitive reactions and many other factors are also involved. Research has led to a number of drugs being developed, most of them highly effective but also extremely expensive, as manufacture is complicated. One might think that rheumatic conditions would pose less of a threat as a result and indeed be less common, but in fact the opposite is the case. The reason for this is that the drugs used treat only the symptoms and not the underlying cause. Some of these drugs are excellent, and will rapidly relieve and even completely remove pain; others will just as rapidly deal with inflammation and the pain caused by this. Patients will be symptom-free in no time, but unfortunately this cannot be called a state of health.

By contrast, biological therapy aims not only to relieve symptoms but also to achieve a genuine cure. It goes without saying that this is a much harder task.

Diet is a major factor. The basic rules are: no pork, and as far as possible a vegetarian diet low in salt and protein; get rid of excess weight by reducing food intake as required. Sometimes the whole metabolism is too much on the acid side. In that case, Basic will help or a mixture of bases.

Experience has shown that beekeepers rarely suffer from rheumatic complaints; this is due to the fact that they are regularly stung by bees. There is a long tradition of using the venom of bees and ants in natural rheumatism therapy. In the past, people suffering from such conditions would simply allow themselves to be stung by bees, use spirit of ants or even take their courage in both hands and sit down in a clump of nettles (which contain a 'poison' similar to that of bees and ants) and they would be cured. Modern patients are unlikely to submit to such heroic measures, however effective. Fortunately numerous preparations containing bee and ant venom are available, among them Apis/Bryonia and Equisetum/Formica. Preparations made from nettle leaves are also available. A herbal product with a base of goat's grease is Caprisana ointment. Traumeel® is widely available as ointment, drops, tablets or for injection.

Internally, take Rheumadoron 102A, 10–15 drops three times daily. A useful homeopathic medicine is Harpagophytum 3x as tablets or, even more effective, injections.

Teas are extremely helpful if taken for an extended period, especially if they contain birch leaves (for instance, Weleda Rheuma Tea); take two cups daily. Weleda Birch Elixir serves the same purpose. Tea mixtures containing grapple plant (devil's claw = Harpagophytum) have also proved helpful.

Most of these natural products will give rapid relief, but what really matters is their alterative action, so that the disease is gradually overcome. Other alterative measures are moor baths and mud packs, many of which are available at continental spas specializing in rheumatic conditions. To some extent it is also possible to carry these treatments out at home and products are available for this purpose. All medicated baths are contraindicated in the acute inflammatory stage.

Gout

Gout, which is nowadays listed among rheumatic conditions, has recently shown a marked increase. There can be no doubt but that this is partly due to increased meat consumption. The result is that uric acid crystals are deposited in various joints, especially in the big toe.

It is obvious that a meat-free diet will be essential. Getting rid of the uric acid is helped by producing sweats, keeping warm generally and drinking plenty of mineral water. On the European Continent, certain mineral waters such as Wernarzer and Fachinger are considered especially suitable. Alcohol should be completely avoided and excess weight reduced. There are medicines which reduce the production of uric acid. They are very effective, but only for so long as they are taken. Apart from this the treatment is the same as for chronic rheumatism, taking in addition Mandragora comp., 15–20 drops three times daily.

Arthritis

Chronic degenerative joint diseases that do not involve inflammation require different treatment, although some of the preparations suggested for the treatment of rheumatic conditions may also be used. Arthritis affects above all the knee joint. Processes of this kind (deposits, concretions, degeneration of cartilage) may also develop in the shoulder joint, which gradually becomes stiff and painful. In this case, regular daily exercise is the most effective treatment, with the range of movement extended a little each day, a few minutes at a time. Medication and ointments as above.

As with all conditions affecting the joints or spine, overweight makes the situation much worse. A reduction in body weight often brings remarkable relief.

Herbal preparations to be taken by mouth are widely available. Externally, Arnica comp./Formica ointment, may be applied. If the usually chronic condition becomes acute and there is increased pain, Harpagophytum 3x (one tablet every two hours) can be helpful.

Spinal disease, back problems

These may involve the same kind of degenerative changes as in arthritis, in which case one speaks of spondylarthritis. Connective tissue weakness may also cause intervertebral disk prolapse ('slipped disk'). Back problems are often due to wrong posture (for instance, at work), the wrong kind of shoes (high heels) and so on. It will often need years of treatment to correct such changes. The wrong kind of stress on the cervical spine (in the neck) may cause headaches. Spastic conditions of the muscles in the neck and back are very common today and on their part limit free movement of the spine even further. It is not surprising, therefore, to find that spinal conditions are on the increase.

A doctor must be consulted to establish the exact cause and condition. At the same time, care must be taken to remove stresses of the kind described and aim for harmony of movement (swimming, walking, eurythmy). It is a matter of self-discipline. Many sports (especially competitive sports) tend to cause increased muscle spasm.

A range of Disci comp. preparations have been developed that can be prescribed for these disorders; they are available as pilules, ointments and injections. The choice of preparation depends on the diagnosis, for instance, Disci comp. cum Argento if nerve function is also impaired, or Disci/Viscum comp. cum Stanno for calcification and malformation. These preparations are most effective if given by injection.

Examples of the many compound homoeopathic preparations are Chirofossat® and Araniforce® and Hocura®-Spondylose ointment.

Muscle spasm may be relieved by taking a bath to which one or two tablespoons of 20% copper sulphate solution have been added (37–38°C, 99–100°F, 15–20 minutes, with the back of the head immersed).

Infections

Abscesses, boils

Warm, almost hot compresses with a decoction of fenugreek seeds (Trigonella foenum-graecum) are helpful.

Apply Mercurialis perennis 10% ointment around but not on the focal point and cover with a gauze dressing. Medicines to be taken depend on the situation, as follows. If an abscess cannot be prevented, Hepar sulphuris 4x, 1 tablet (or pinch of powder) five times daily for one or two days, will help to resolve it. If the infection is still in its early stage, however, an attempt may be made to 'disperse' it, using Hepar sulphuris 12x.

Myristica sebifera 4x, 7 drops hourly or five times a day, is known as the 'homeopathic knife' and helps the pus to be discharged. Take Silicea 12x once the abscess has opened, and 5x when it is in its final stage, 1 tablet (or pinch of powder) five times daily.

Influenza (flu) and feverish colds

Influenza is today considered to be a virus infection. Yet some people are known to be more susceptible to infection than others. Influenza vaccines confer only limited protection, firstly because it cannot be known in advance which virus will be responsible for the next epidemic and secondly because it is far from certain how long the protection will last.

The phrase 'catching a cold' points to one cause — susceptible individuals are often found to have an imbalance

in their heat metabolism. Heat loss makes people more susceptible to infection. It should be said, however, that anyone who is really healthy is unlikely to catch a cold and can
afford to get chilled without having to suffer the consequences. Susceptibility is a sign of an inner disorder, even
if this is not immediately apparent. Disorders, or weak-
nesses, of heat metabolism are common today; they may be
due to unsuitable clothing, or indeed to lack of exercise. An
obvious symptom are the permanently cold feet (and
hands) one sees with so many chronic diseases. This kind
of disorder often proves an obstacle to effective treatment.
It is best treated with alternating hot and cold foot baths
(see p.27). Many people also have poor resistance because
of a poor diet (see p.22f) or frequent suppression of acute
illnesses. Continuous stress may also have this effect. Continuous stress may also have this effect, as well as fear. The
expression 'getting cold feet' points to this.

Susceptible individuals often develop influenza after
getting thoroughly chilled. The natural method of dealing
with this is to get really warm by taking a hot bath, a sauna,
or the like. Otherwise the body will try and do this by producing a fever. The rise in temperature first makes the individual shiver, often followed by rigors. These are signs
that the body is trying to overcome the chill by producing
more heat. Please note, however, that a hot bath, while extremely useful in preventing a cold or influenza developing, is contraindicated once the body temperature starts to
rise.

Whilst a 'common' cold tends to begin with being thoroughly chilled, its end is often marked by a sweat, indicating that the body is now generating sufficient heat. By
providing heat in good time, using measures that will also
produce a sweat, it is therefore possible to prevent the illness or at least shorten it.

Such a healthy sweat must be distinguished from the

cold sweat that may develop in its acute form if there is cardiovascular weakness and may be a real torment, especially at night. It is often due to being over stimulated; these individuals cannot 'let go', sleep is shallow and interrupted. Half a teaspoonful of Conchae 5% (not a sleeping drug!) taken at night may help here, or Weleda Calcium Supplement 2, 1 teaspoonful at night. Sage tea washes have also proved effective. Salvysat contains a concentrated extract of sage leaves (20 drops or 1 or 2 tablets three times daily). Night sweats may also occur with rheumatic conditions, gout or tuberculosis, when different treatment is required.

Medication designed to bring down a fever — pills, tablets, suppositories and so on, that is, the majority of 'influenza remedies' — must be avoided. A temperature is the body's natural method of overcoming the disease. Experience has shown that it is far better to stay in bed for three to five days. The rapid improvement achieved with drugs tends to be followed by months, if not years, of being only 'half alive' and never feeling entirely well.

The body's efforts are supported by hot lemon drinks, to which Melissa comp. may be added.

Natural sources of vitamin C that have always proved useful in the prevention of influenza include lemon, sea buckthorn juice (available as Sandthorn Elixir) and acerola (based on a cherry with unusually high vitamin C content). At the time of the year when influenza is most likely to strike, keeping warm and the use of applied heat, for instance, in a sauna, give added protection.

Another way to improve resistance is with medicines that act as alteratives, for example a combination of Thuja 2x, Baptisia tinct. rad. 2x and Echinacea rad. 3x. This may also be taken after a bout of influenza to help convalescence.

One of the most effective homeopathic treatments in the

early stages of colds, influenza and other feverish illnesses, is Aconitum napellus 4x, 5 drops at hourly intervals, or, even better, in the compound preparation Infludo, taken as directed, hourly to begin with. Gelsemium 4x or 6x helps to relieve headaches and aching limbs. At the beginning of the century, Professor Bier, a German surgeon with an international reputation who was much in favour of homeopathy and natural medicine, suggested putting a single drop of tincture of iodine (obtainable from chemists) in a glass of water and taking regular sips of this over a number of hours. This stimulates the natural defences and will in most cases stop an attack of influenza or a cold that is still in its early stage. Please note that the effect is not due to disinfectant properties of iodine, and nothing but simple tincture of iodine should be used.

Infludo is indicated with every type of influenza. It is a combination of homeopathic potencies based on anthroposophical principles and promotes healing and whole body reactions over a wide spectrum. As soon as the first symptoms appear, take 7–10 drops hourly (or put 50 drops in half a glass of water and take regular sips over a five-hour period). Gradually increase the time intervals as symptoms get less, finally taking the drops only three times daily until fully recovered. Some individuals are over-stimulated by Infludo so that they feel overexcited and cannot go to sleep. They should take Ferrum phosphoricum comp. instead, 10–15 pilules hourly; this is also better for children.

For children, suppositories of Belladonna comp., Chamomilla comp., or Aconitum/China comp. may be used once or several times daily. They do not contain chemicals that suppress a fever, but help the body's efforts to heal itself. Elderflower tea to which freshly squeezed lemon juice is added supports the treatment. 15–20 drops of Melissa comp. may also be added, and the tea may be sweetened, preferably with honey.

The immune defences may be strengthened by giving an extract of Echinacea (purple coneflower or Rudbeckia), a North American plant which may also be found in many European gardens or grown by pharmaceutical firms. Echinacin® is probably the most established and well-known product. Suitably prepared, the plant can be shown to activate white blood cells, increasing their numbers, strengthening the immune system. Susceptibility to colds does indeed indicate a weakness in the immune system. To stimulate it, we have to take note of what is said under Exercise. A stimulus may be too weak or too powerful. In either case the interval between exercises is as important as the exercises themselves. Continuous stimulation causes stress. Where medicines are concerned this means that 'a lot does not help a lot!' This may not be a new principle but it is often ignored. For the medicines we have mentioned it means, quite generally, that those that provide a stimulus should only be given at onset, that is when one gets a chill and has a rising temperature. They should not be used when the condition has reached a high point and there is a high temperature. In that case, it is better to have one of the above-mentioned compound homoeopathic preparations.

With prevention, too, it is advisable to stop treatment for half a week after taking the medication for a week or so, or to have one week's break after two week's treatment, and so on. The intervals may be lengthened after a time.

It is also possible to stimulate the immune system with an extract of Eleutherococcus root from the Siberian taiga. A number of firms produce this. The plant is related to ginseng and is a general tonic.

Alterative measures are needed for individuals who have frequent attacks of influenza. It may be enough just to limit protein intake, which generally tends to be too high anyway. Fresh foods should be taken (not to be confused with a raw-food diet that consists of nothing but raw foods). Part of the diet should be raw, for instance, some of the vegetables eaten as a salad. Give fresh muesli daily, made by soaking 2 or 3 tablespoons of absolutely freshly ground grains (wheat, barley or oats, on their own or mixed) in water for about twelve hours and then adding grated or chopped apple, banana to replace sugar, fruits of the season and cream.

Applied heat (hot baths, sauna, producing a sweat) are the foundation stone of alterative therapy. Medicinal baths may also be indicated, with Rosemary Bath Milk added to stimulate heat production, Oleum Pini sylvest. if there is a tendency to develop bronchitis, coryza and so on.

After some time, the body should be hardened, that is, it needs to be trained with the aid of cold water applications (see p.26).

The reasons for repeated attacks of influenza are many and varied; common causes include acute diseases that have not been completely overcome, continuous stress, above all nervous strain, dietary faults or constitutional problems. It is necessary to consult a doctor to establish the cause.

Very often it is a matter of poor resistance or a weakness of the immune system, which again may be due to a number of causes. A high quality wholefood diet is advisable. Medicines that help in this direction are Echinacea 30%, 20 drops three times daily for 2–3 months. When the risk is acute, change to the Thuja 2x, Baptisia rad. 2x and Echinacea rad. 3x combination, 20 drops or 1 tablet several times daily.

Supportive measures may be needed to deal with cough, bronchitis and coryza (see under those headings).

Gynaecological conditions

These disorders may be due to many different causes and medical advice should be sought. A few of the more common problems are discussed below. All women, even if in good health, should go for regular medical check-ups.

Problems with periods

A basic medicament designed to establish regular rhythms without forcing or suppressing nature, is Menodoron, a product combining several medicinal plants. Take 10–15 drops three times daily for at least three months, but not during periods. This not only helps to establish a regular monthly cycle but usually also relieves the pain and discomfort of periods.

Irregularities in the second stage of the cycle (corpus luteus hormone production) leading to frequent and excessive bleeding, respond to combinations like the following: Agnus castus 2x, Caulophyllum 5x, Ignatia 7x, Lilium tigr. 4x. If the problem lies in the first stage of the cycle (oestrogen production), Cimicifuga 3x or 6x, 8 drops three times daily, may prove helpful.

Premenstrual syndrome or tension responds well to a combination such as Lupulinum 9x, Condurango 4x, Cyclamen 5x, Iris 3x. Dosages are given on the packs. A useful dietary supplement is Evening Primrose Oil (see p.46).

Period pain (dysmenorrhoea)

Take Menodoron (see above) between periods, and 10–15 pilules of Belladonna/Chamomilla several times daily as the period starts. The pilules may also be taken in alternation with Potentilla anserina 2x.

Vaginal discharge (leucorrhoea)

It will be necessary to establish the cause, for local treatment is unlikely to clear this up. Occasionally the condition is due to the wrong kind of hygiene, that is, douches containing irritant substances, or getting chilled, e.g. because of not being dressed warmly enough. Warm sitz baths (not full baths) with marjoram and balm (Melissa officinalis) tea.

Menopause (climacteric)

Hot flushes are common during the change. A mixture like the following has been found helpful: Cimicifuga 6x, Sepia 6x, Lachesis 6x, Ignatia 6x, Sanguinaria 6x; take 1 or 2 tablets three times daily for about three months. Depending on the individual constitution, Ovarium comp., a pinch of powder three times daily, or Sepia comp., 10 drops three times daily, may be indicated. Cimicifuga 3x or 6x may also be indicated.

Mental upsets, overexertion or excessive stimulation with coffee or tea are known to make the symptoms worse. Salt has a similar effect. It is therefore advisable to reduce the intake of these. Salvysat, a concentrated sage extract, may be used for hot flushes (1 or 2 tablets three times daily).

Pregnancy

Fuller details on how to approach pregnancy, questions of diet and other related problems may be found in *A Guide to Child Health* by Glöckler and Goebel.

For morning sickness: Nausyn, one tablet several times daily for 2–4 weeks.

To stimulate the calcium metabolism of mother and child: Weleda Calcium Supplement 1 and 2; from the fourth month onwards, a pinch of the powder or 1 tablet of No.1 in the mornings, No.2 at night.

For varicose veins and venous stasis (see also under Varicose veins), apply Weleda Skin Tone Lotion once or twice a day, especially to the lower legs, using gentle stroking movements. Also take a preparation containing horse chestnut extract 100 mg (coated tablets usually contain 20 mg of aescin, 1 ml of the drops 40 mg) or baths with Weleda or Wala Aesculus Bath Lotion added. For leg cramps at night take a pinch of powder or 1 tablet of Cuprum arsen. 6x at night or several times daily.

To prevent stretch marks (striae), massage regularly and carefully with Weleda Massage Oil.

Lactation: Weleda Lactagogue Tea, one or two cups a day, and Oleum Lactagogum, gently massaged into the breasts twice a day, are useful for bringing on the milk.

Breastfeeding mothers should continue to take Weleda Calcium Supplements 1 and 2 on a regular basis, also Weleda Blackthorn Elixir.

Children

Infant care

Mothers knew instinctively how to do things in the past. Today the old methods have either been forgotten or are considered doubtful.

Good infant care starts during pregnancy, which may be a natural state but nevertheless needs special attention (see Lockie *The Family Guide to Homoeopathy*). An expectant mother who smokes, harms not only herself but also her child. The same applies to drinking alcohol and taking other stimulants. It does not need major scientific investigations to see the harm done; ordinary common sense makes it quite clear.

Giving birth is itself a natural process. The less outside intervention, the better it is usually for the child — except where there are complications, of course. But we should at least make sure that the delivery room is warm enough; if not, the child, coming from an environment where the temperature was 37°C (99°F), suffers a shock.

Bathing the baby every day is a bad habit we have got into nowadays. Infants do of course have to be kept clean, but they need a bath only once or twice a week.

It is now generally accepted that breast-feeding is the best form of nutrition for an infant. Even the most 'perfect' recipe for a bottle feed, containing all the nutrients corresponding to mother's milk, cannot replace it. If bottle-feeding is the only option, the aim should be to make it as natural as possible. In this respect, ordinary pasteurized milk is far superior to UHT milk. Pasteurized organic milk is now available from some supermarkets and is definitely preferable. Products containing condensed milk should be completely avoided. If ready-made mixtures have to be used, those based on dried milk are preferable.

Prepared bottle feeds are made with milk and cereal products. Demeter quality Holle Baby Foods are specially recommended. The amounts and number of feeds to be given are stated on the packs; they depend on the child's age. Detailed information on feeding is given in *A Guide to Child Health* by Glöckler and Goebel.

With supplementary feeding and the change to solids the principle is the same as for every wholefood diet: foods must be 'living' if they are to be life-giving. The closer they are to life, that is, the fresher and less processed they are, the better. Methods used in the preparation of food should not be designed to kill and isolate specific substances but to maintain and enhance the vitality of the food. In general we may say that the greater the chemical changes made to a food the less its value (see also p.22).

Good infant care also calls for the right attitude to children. They are not adults, but entirely different by nature. Young children are great imitators and what the grown-ups do is much more important than what they say. Up to their seventh year, children take in the actions of adults and reproduce them exactly.

Developmental disorders of childhood include **rickets** which is generally treated with vitamin D today. The vitamin is also used to prevent rickets, but it has been shown that it is in fact a hormone and certainly not as harmless as other vitamins. Vitamin D promotes calcification and can therefore cure rickets. In children who do not have rickets, however, it will still encourage calcification and cause excessive hardening.

Biological rickets prevention consists in making sure that the child gets sufficient light. In most cases being under a blue sky is all that is needed. Special preparations developed to provide a high degree of protection from rickets are Apatite/Phosphorus comp. and Conchae/Quercus comp., both available in two varieties — S for infants and K for young children. The dose is 1 or 2 times 5 drops of Apatite/ Phosphorus comp. in water in the mornings, and 1–2 pinches of Conchae/Quercus comp. powder at night. These preparations do not confer complete protection, and the children should be under medical supervision.

Night starts are fairly common in young children. They will suddenly start to cry an hour or two after going to sleep and there is no apparent reason. They will often not even recognize their parents. This is basically a harmless phenomenon, but it may happen again and again for weeks or even years. In most cases, Bryophyllum Argento cultum 1%, 5 drops in water once or twice at night, will prove effective. In other cases, particularly if it is more a case of **sleepwalking**, Stramonium 15x, 5–10 drops at night, will help. The usual sedatives or sleeping drugs are ineffective and in fact should never be given to children.

For some years it has been observed that infants can suffer from sleeplessness. Naturally, if the parents are restless this can affect the child, but there are families where everything is peaceful and the childcare is fine, but the infant nevertheless lies awake or cries for hours. In the past it was known that some children simply cry for hours. Provided that no cause for the crying can be found by a doctor, parents should not be worried about this. Sedatives should not be given under any ciurcumstances.

Childhood diseases

Essentially these are childhood illnesses involving a high temperature and a red rash — **measles, scarlet fever** and **German measles**. They are an important aspect of full development, for they not only stimulate resistance and strengthen the immune system but also help with mental and inner development. In the past, mothers immediately knew what to do in such cases. Natural therapy consists in avoiding all unnecessary treatment. It is important that the temperature should never be brought down by forcible measures. If it gets extremely high, it will usually be sufficient to apply compresses of water at room temperature to the lower legs, adding a small amount of vinegar or lemon juice if desired. If this does not prove sufficient, apply a body compress of water at room temperature a few hours later (for more details, see works cited for *Home Nursing* under *Further Reading*). The diet should consist of fruit juices and fresh fruit. (For Fever, see p.40).

Instead of chemical anti-fever drugs, use Aconitum/ China comp., suppositories — for children — and pilules (Wala). These do not reduce the fever the way drugs do, but stimulate the natural defences. Additional homeopathic medication depends more on the patient's condition than on the name of the disease. Generally speaking, children with measles often require Aconitum napellus 4x, those with scarlet fever are more likely to need Belladonna 4x; in either case 5 drops five times daily in a small amount of fluid.

The much dreaded complications, especially of measles, are more likely to develop if unsuitable therapeutic measures are taken (for instance, anti-fever drugs).

In rare instances there can be febrile convulsions. While this looks dramatic, in most cases they have passed by the time medical help has been sought. Such convulsions can happen during the time of the increase of the fever, but not at the time of its maximum. For this reason anti-fever drugs are inappropriate. However, if the convulsions last for longer periods, or are repeated, the doctor should be consulted.

Age-related problems

Ageing is a natural process that cannot be stopped, though it may come prematurely or take the wrong course. Rejuvenation and regeneration treatments will at most slightly delay the inevitable. Individuals can guide the process in the right direction by being active in ways that are suitable for their age. Inner rather than physical activity will keep us young in spirit; exclusively physical activity will keep the body functioning well at the physical level but may actually block activities of the mind and spirit, which can then appear as forgetfulness, disorientation, stubbornness and such like.

In addition, older people need less sleep and less food.

Birch Elixir helps to dissolve and eliminate deposits of waste products — a tablespoonful three times daily in herb tea or water, it also makes an excellent 'spring cure.' Sugar-free Birch Elixir is obtainable in Switzerland (Birkenherb).

Belladonna 6x, 8 drops three times daily before meals for two months, then a month's pause, helps to prevent hardening processes.

Scleron, one tablet twice daily for six weeks, then four weeks' pause, with the whole ten-week pattern repeated several times a year, helps to keep mentally alert and prevents 'calcification' and 'forgetfulness.'

An extract made from the leaves of the ginkgo (maidenhair) tree has proved useful in stimulating the circulation in the region of the head and also the extremities. It can be taken at the same time as the above-mentioned medicaments.

Diabetes

Modern drugs have taken away the fear of this disease but they cannot cure it. Patients will have to take medication to the end of their lives. Diabetics also have to be on a restricted diet. In severe cases, diet and medication have to be very accurately established, generally in hospital, and patients must not change them of their own accord.

Lifestyle again plays a crucial role. Young diabetics in particular are well advised to be physically active. Herbal preparations based on a number of plants may prove beneficial, but a doctor should always be consulted before they are used. Bilberry leaf tea has a long tradition in popular medicine.

Many people living in industrialized countries have a disposition for this disease, which to some degree may also be inherited. They have 'latent' diabetes without being aware of it. The causes are many, and the high sugar and refined flour product consumption of our present age favours the disease.

Cancer

This much feared disease always needs medical treatment, which today largely involves surgery, radiotherapy and/or chemotherapy to remove or kill the cancer cells with their tendency for uncontrollable growth. Decisions as to which methods should be used must be made by a cancer specialist. In addition it is possible to stimulate the body's own defences to counteract the growth tendency of cancer cells.

Many doctors have used mistletoe preparations for this purpose for some years (see Lockie in *Further Reading*). The best known mistletoe preparations are Iscador, Helixor, Iscucin, Abnoba-Viscum and Isorel. They are available on prescription only and doctors can obtain full information from the manufacturers.

Cancer is more than a local condition to be treated locally; it affects the whole organism. The whole life situation of the individual needs to be considered, and changes in lifestyle (see p.22f) and diet are beneficial in support of medical treatment. Liver and intestinal function is impaired with most cancer patients and Epsom salts may be helpful in clearing toxins from the intestinal tract (see p.74).

Smoking and sugar should be completely avoided and protein intake limited. It is better for the diet to be sparse rather than too much.

Afterword

Many doctors and health practitioners are currently using the natural therapies and medicines discussed in this book. The fact is, however, that when people go to see their doctor, they usually expect to be given a prescription that will quickly get rid of the problem. Preference is therefore given to medicines that remove symptoms, and medical and pharmaceutical research has in recent years increasingly concentrated on developing powerful, fast-acting drugs that on the surface seem superior to older methods. The principle of healing, achieving a real cure, tends to be neglected.

There will of course be situations where fast-acting chemical drugs are needed. But it must be remembered that these drugs act at a surface level and do not generally deal with causes. The almost inevitable side effects of such drugs (highlighted by the disastrous effects of thalidomide) has led over the years to a tightening-up of drugs legislation. For even greater safety, the authorities now demand not only stringent drugs tests of general validity but also proof of efficacy. The idea behind this — to provide for greater safety and reliability — seems a good one; unfortunately its implementation has meant that a procedure that is entirely appropriate to chemically produced drugs is also being applied to natural medicines.

One of the main arguments put forward in defence of this testing is that natural medicines can also be harmful. There can be no doubt, of course, that some plants and animals are highly poisonous and may even prove fatal; the required effects are all a matter of dosage and proper use. It is perfectly possible to kill someone with ordinary table salt, by getting them to eat half a pound of it. This same table salt can be very beneficial for people with low blood pressure, for example, and practically poisonous for anyone with high blood pressure. The same applies to coffee and other things that are part of daily life. This demonstrates the problems that arise when criteria are based on 'normal levels,' maximum doses and legal requirements.

Safety legislation is also extending to homeopathic medicines. For that reason some remedies which have poisonous substances in them require a prescription despite the fact that in homeopathic doses it would be practically impossible to be poisoned by them. It is likely that this sort of legislation will extend to other well-tried remedies.

By contrast, there is practically no legislation concerning two clearly damaging substances, namely alcohol and tobacco. While it is not the task of the state to ban all pleasurable substances, this attitude stands in grotesque contrast to the concern and strict legislation of natural remedies.

The ongoing programme of legislation (which also varies from state to state) often causes old tried and tested remedies to be altered in composition or dosage to fit the regulations. This safetly legislation is often deceptive as it forces practitioners to use other cures which — though tested to modern standards — have unknown long-term side effects.

With natural medicines, the principles of use are quite different. The preparations mentioned in this book are made from plants, animal substances or minerals (phytotherapy, naturopathy, homeopathy, anthroposophical medicine) and none of them have toxic effects if used according to directions. The action of these medicines is not primarily to deal with an isolated symptom but to stimulate the organism so that it can overcome the disease.

Suppression of diseases with drugs that remove symptoms is widespread today. The consequences are that the numbers of sick people are constantly increasing and costs are rising at an alarming rate in the health (or rather 'sickness') sector, where the limits of capacity have almost been reached. Regulations to reduce costs will not change the situation; on the contrary, costs will escalate further, as such regulations address the symptoms and not the root cause. Additional problems are due to misguided preventive measures. The suppression and prevention of diseases tends to cause a shift to other, generally more serious diseases. With 'health' systems such as the National Health Service in the United Kingdom and private insurance, people want to 'get their money's worth,' and the issuing of sickness certificates to people who are not expected to make any effort of their own, leads many to feel almost that they have a right to sickness. Individuals who systematically ruin their health — by smoking, alcohol abuse and sheer neglect, for instance — are not only acting irresponsibly where they themselves and their families are concerned but also causing a loss to the community at large by being a drain on the agencies that provide the resources for medical care.

We cannot expect to change the situation by bringing in even more stringent laws and government regulations, for it is the system itself that is sick. Fundamental change will have to depend on the insight and initiative of every individual. We need to understand the meaning of individual illnesses, do what is necessary to achieve a real cure and broaden our lifestyle by introducing the different types of hygiene that have been referred to in the introductory chapters. Then and only then will healing be possible, so that illness is truly overcome and health achieved.

Appendix

Beyond the level of home remedies described in this book, anthroposophical medicine is practised in the UK and elsewhere by a number of doctors. In the UK, consultation and treatment are available both through the NHS and privately. For information, contact:

The Anthroposophical Medical Association, Park Attwood, Trimpley, Bewdley, DY12 1RE.

Suggestions for a medicine chest

Every home should have a medicine chest or cupboard for providing first aid and coping with minor ailments. Of course this kind of care at home can never substitute for your doctor's professional care and advice.

The medicine chest or cupboard should be fitted with a lockable compartment for storing medicaments. There should also be a drawer for bandages, dressings and other first aid equipment.

The medicine chest must of course be kept somewhere out of reach of children, and preferably in a cool, dry place. All medicines must be labelled to show their contents and directions for use.

Strong medicines that have been prescribed by your doctor for a particular case of illness should not normally be kept after the illness is over. Ask your doctor if they can be kept for future use.

Basic equipment should include the nursing aids that will be frequently needed, an adequate supply of dressings, and a range of herb teas and medicines that your doctor has prescribed.

Don't forget to list your doctor's telephone number, together with the local hospital/clinic or other emergency services.

The medicine chest must always be fully stocked and ready for use. Be sure to replace medicines and dressings as soon as they have been used.

Household remedies

Laxative tea	for constipation
Valerian	for nervous restlessness (not if there is a temperature)
Fennel tea	for stomach upsets of young children
Peppermint tea	for stomach upsets of adults
Camomile tea	for spasms, colic, inflammation
Lime blossom tea	for colds
Sage tea	for sore throats
Wormwood tea	for weak digestion
Melissa comp.	for general indisposition
Olbas Oil/ Japanese Peppermint Oil	for colds, local inflammation, pain

Medicines

The numbers given after the medicines in the following list refer to the pages of this book where the problem is discussed.

Mercurialis comp. Ointment	Wounds (p.34)
Combudoron Lotion and Ointment	Burns (p.35f)
Arnica Lotion	Injuries (external) (p.35)
Infludo	Influenza (p.88f)
Cardiodoron A	Cardiovascular system (p.63f)
Veratrum album 4x	Circulation (p.71)
Carbo Coffeae (Coffee charcoal)	Diarrhoea (p.71)
Artemisia comp.	Sensation of fullness (p.69)
Mercurius cyanatus 4x	Purulent sore throat (p.58)
Bolus Eucalypti comp.	Sore throat (p.58f)
Carbo Betulae comp.	Gastroenteritis (p.71f)
Chamomilla comp. suppositories	Children with a temperature (p.91)
Levisticum (Radix) 3x/Levisticum 10% oil	Earache/Middle ear inflammation (p.54)

Equipment, nursing aids
Hot water bottle
Irrigator for enemas
Thermometer
Scissors
Splinter forceps
Tongue depressor
Safety pins
Leather fingerstall

First aid materials
2 gauze bandages, 6 cm (2¼") wide
2 gauze bandages, 8 cm (3") wide
1 first aid dressing, small
1 first aid dressing, medium
1 sterile wound dressing, 50 x 4 cm (20" x 1½") (non-adhesive)
1 sterile wound dressing, 50 x 6 cm (20" x 2¼") (non-adhesive)
1 sterile wound, 50 x 8 cm (20" x 3") (non-adhesive)
2 bandage clips
1 triangular bandage

List of medicines

Where homeopathic medicines are listed as 2x or 4x, the 6x potency, more common in Britain, may be safely used if the 4x is not available. For this English edition, they have been limited to products listed in *Martindale's Extra Pharmacopoeia.*

The addresses of manufacturers are given on p.119f. Medicines may be obtained directly from the manufacturers if your local pharmacist or health food store does not stock them.

Further information for the medical profession is obtainable from Weleda (UK) Ltd, Heanor Road, Ilkeston, Derbyshire DE7 8DR.

Names of products may vary a little in different countries. Where the name is recognizably similar, it is not specially noted. Where the product is available under a different name in New Zealand (NZ) or in South Africa (SA) it is shown.

Abbreviations:

HFS   Health Food or Wholefood Store
Hom.   homeopathic medicine
(o)   needs to be specially ordered
POM   available on a doctor's prescription only.
       These indications may vary in different countries.

Name of product	*Supplier or Manufacturer*
ABC Liniment	HFS
Abnoba-Visum®	POM
Aconitum/China comp. Suppositories and Pilules (NZ use Chamomilla comp. suppositories, Weleda NZ)	Wala
Aconitum comp. Oleum	Wala
Aconitum napellus 4x	Hom.
Aesculus Bath Lotion	Wala
Allium cepa 3x	Hom.
Amara Drops (NZ Amara bitters)	Weleda
Anaemodoron/Gentian (SA Enzian-Anaemodoron)	Weleda
Anise/Pyrites	Weleda
Apatite/Phosphorus comp. (NZ Apis/ Belladona/Echinacea/Levisticum 3x)	Weleda
Apis/Bryonia	Wala
Apis 3x	Hom.
Archangelica comp. Ointment	Weleda
Argentum 0.4% Ointment	Weleda

Arnica 3x, 20x	Hom.
Arnica comp./Formica Ointment	Weleda
Arnica Essence	Wala
Arnica Lotion	Weleda
Arsenicum album 10x	Hom.
Artemisia comp.	Weleda (SA)
Avena sativa/Valeriana	Weleda
Avena sativa comp.	
(NZ Avena comp. sedative drops)	Weleda
Balsamicum Ointment	Weleda
Barium iodatum 4x	Hom.
Bearberry leaves	Herbalists
Belladonna/Chamomilla	Wala
(NZ use Chamomilla/Nicotiana comp.,	Weleda NZ)
Belladonna 4x, 6x	Hom.
Belladonna comp. Suppositories	Wala
Berberis fruit, Ointment 10%	HFS, Herbalists
Bidor® (SA Kephalodoron)	Weleda
Birch Elixir	Weleda
Birkenherb®	Weleda (SA)
Blackthorn Elixir (SA Shlehen Elixir,	
NZ use Prunus Elixir)	Weleda
Bolus Eucalypti comp.	Weleda
Borago 20% Lotion	Weleda
Bryophyllum Argento cultum 1%	Weleda
Calamus Oil	Wala
Calcium Supplement 1 and 2	
(SA Aufbaukalkland 2)	Weleda
Calendula/Stibium Ointment®	Weleda
Calendula Essence	Wala
Calendula Lotion	Weleda
Camomile Ointment (SA)	Weleda
Cantharis 10x	Hom.
Cantharis comp.	Wala
Caprisana Ointment/Sidroga	HFS
Carbo Betulae 5%/Oleum aeth. Carvi 1%	
(SA Carvon Tablets)	Weleda
Carbo Coffeae (SA)	Weleda
Cardiodoron® A	Weleda
(NZ For jet lag also: Aurum/Cardiodoron, Weleda NZ)	

Cardiomax Garlic Perles	Höfel's/HFS
Carduus marianus	Weleda
Catarrh Cream	Weleda
Ceratum Ratanhia comp.	Weleda (o)
Chamomilla comp. Suppositories	Weleda
Chamomilla matricaria Root 3x	Weleda
Choleodoron®	Weleda
Cimicifuga 3x, 6x	Hom.
Cinnabar 6x	Weleda
Clairo Tea	Weleda
Clorets	Chemists
Coldastop (SA)	HFS
Combudoron® Gel, Lotion, Ointment	Weleda
Conchae/Quercus comp.	Weleda
Crataegus Drops, Tablets	Weleda
Cuprum aceticum 4x	Hom.
Cuprum arsen. 6x	Hom.
Cuprum met. 0.4% Ointment (SA)	Weleda
Cuprum met prep. Ointment	Weleda
Dermatodoron®	Weleda
Digestodoron®	Weleda
Disci comp.	Wala
Drosera 6x	Weleda
Dual-Lax	G.R.Lane/HFS
Echinacea 30% (NZ Echinacea/Thuja comp.)	Weleda
Echinacea Mouth Spray	Wala
Epsom salts	Chemists
Equisetum/Formica	Wala
Equisetum 4x, 15x	Hom.
Equisetum cum Sulphure tostum 3x, trit.	Weleda
Equisetum Tea	Weleda
Eucalyptus oil (Oleum Pini sylvest.)	Wala
Ferrum per Urtica 1% (NZ Ferrum Ustum comp.)	Weleda
Ferrum phosphoricum comp.	Weleda (o)
Fink Cysto Capsules	HFS
Gelsemium 4x, 6x	Hom.
Gencydo®	Weleda
Gentiana lutea 5%	Weleda
Harpagophytum	Duenner/HFS

Hawthorn (Crataegus)	Gerard/HFS
Helixor®	POM
Hepar/Magnesium 4x	Weleda
Hepar/Stannum 4x	Weleda
Hepar sulphuris 4x, 12x	Hom.
Hepatodoron®	Weleda
Holle Baby Foods	HFS
Ignatia 6x	Weleda
Infludo® (NZ use Agropyron comp. or Echinacea/Thuja comp.)	Weleda
Ipecacuanha 6x	Hom.
Iscador®	POM
Iscucin®	POM
Isorel®	POM
Japanese Peppermint Oil	Obbekjaer's/HFS
Juglans regia 1x	Weleda
Kalium phosphoricum comp.	Weleda
Kieserite 4x, 6x, 20x	Weleda
Lachesis 12x dil.	Hom.
Lactisol	Wirt/HFS
Lavender Bath Milk	Weleda
Laxadoron (SA Clairo Tablets)	Weleda
Levisticum 10% Oil	Weleda
Levisticum radix 3x	Weleda
Lichenes comp. (SA)	Weleda
Magnesium phos. 3x, 6x	Hom.
Mallow Oil	Wala
Mandragora comp.	Weleda
Melissa comp.	Weleda
Menodoron®	Weleda
Mercurialis comp. Ointment	Wala
Mercurialis perennis Ointment 10%	Weleda
Mercurius cyanatus 4x	Hom.
Mercurius vivus nat. 6x	Weleda
Myristica sebifera 4x	Hom.
Nausyn®	POM
Nelsons Hay Fever Tablets HFS,	Chemists
Nux vomica 4x	Hom.

Olbas Oil	G.R.Lane/HFS
(SA Herbaforce, Weleda SA)	
Oleum lactagogum	Weleda
Oleum Rhinale I and II	Weleda
Ortisan/Ortis	HFS
Ovarium comp.	Wala
Oxalis comp.	Weleda
Pertudoron 1 and 2	
(NZ use Resina Laricis comp. inh.)	Weleda
Petasites comp. cum Veronica	Wala
Petasites comp. cum Quercu	Wala
Phytovarix Massage Gel	Arkopharma
Pine Bath Milk	Weleda
Pinella Tea	
(SA Species Stomachicae Digestion Tea)	Weleda
Pneumonium LA	Wala
Potentilla anserina 2x	Hom.
Potter's Balm of Gilead Cough Mixture	Potters/HFS
Potters Comfrey Ointment	HFS
(SA Weleda Symphytum 10% Ointment)	Weleda SA
Pumilio or Dwarf Pine Oil	HFS
Quercus 1x	Weleda
Renodoron®	Weleda
Rheumadoron 102A	Weleda
Robinia comp.	Wala
Rosemary Bath Milk	Weleda
Sandthorn Elixir (SA)	Weleda
Scleron®	Weleda
Secale/Quartz	Wala
Senokot	Chemists
Sepia comp.	Weleda
Silicea 5x, 12x	Hom.
Silicea comp.	Wala
Solum oliginosum comp. Pilules and	
Bath Lotion	Wala
Stibium met. prep. 6x Powder	
(NZ Marmor/Stibium 6x)	Weleda
Stramonium 15x	Hom.
Sytra Tea	Weleda

Tanacetum (SA) Strath,	Cedar
Thuja occidentalis 4x	Hom.
Thuja Argento cultum 0.1%	Weleda
Veratrum album 4x	Hom.
Veronica officinalis 1x (NZ Veronica 10%)	Weleda
Vick's Vapour Rub	Chemists
Vitamin D	Cantassium/HFS
Wala Acne Treatment	Wala
Wala Nerve Food (SA)	Wala
Wala Nose Balm, Nose Balm Mild	Wala
WCS Powder	Weleda
Weleda Cough Drops	Weleda
Weleda Cough Elixir	Weleda
Weleda Gargle and Mouthwash	Weleda
Weleda Herbal Toothpaste	Weleda
Weleda Kidney Tea	Weleda
Weleda Lactagogue Tea	Weleda
Weleda Massage Oil	Weleda
Weleda Rheuma Tea	Weleda
Weleda Salt Toothpaste	Weleda
Weleda Sedative Tea	Weleda
Weleda Skin Tone Lotion	Weleda

Manufacturers and distributors

Anthroposophical medicines
Great Britain: Weleda (UK) Ltd
Heanor Road, Ilkeston, DE7 8DR, Great Britain
Tel. 0115 944 8222   Fax 0115-944 8210
www.weleda.co.uk   Email: Info@Weleda.co.uk
Wala products distributed by Weleda (UK) Ltd

Ireland: Weleda (Irl.) Ltd
Scoughan, Blessington, Co. Wicklow, Ireland
Tel. 045-865 575   Fax 045-865 827

United States: Weleda Inc,
PO Box 249, Congers, NY 10920, U S A
Tel. 914-268 8572   Fax 914-268 8574
Email: Info@Weleda.com

Canada: Purity Life Health Products Ltd
6 Commerce Street, Acton, Ont. L71 2X3, Canada
Tel. 519-853 3511   Fax 519-853 4660

Australia: Weleda Pty Ltd
488 Burke Street, Melbourne VIC 3000, Australia
Tel. 03-9723 7278

New Zealand: Weleda New Zealand Ltd
PO Box 8132, Havelock North, New Zealand
Tel. 96-877 7394   Fax 96-877 4989
Email: customerservices@weleda.co.nz

South Africa: Weleda SA
PO Box 5502, Johannesburg 2000, South Africa
Tel. 011-444 6921   Fax 011-444 8774
Email: eleanor@Pharma.co.za

Homeopathic medicines only
A. Nelson & Co
    5 Endeavour Way, London SW19 9UH
    Tel. 020-8946 8527
Ainsworth's Homoeopathic Pharmacy
    38 New Cavendish Street, London W1
    Tel. 020-7935 5330 or 7486 0459

Herbal and general health products
The following UK suppliers will supply direct if Health
Food Stores cannot order:

Arkopharma, Hindhead, Surrey GU26 6AA
Cantassium, 225 Putney Bridge Road, London SW5 2PY
Dr Duenner AG, Kirchberg, Switzerland
Gerard House Ltd, 3 Wickham Road, Boscombe,
    Bournemouth BH7 6TX
Hoefel's products: Distributed by Fords Ltd, Marfleet, Hull
    HU9 5NJ
G.R. Lane Health Products Ltd, Gloucester
Obbekjaer's Oil of Peppermint: Distributed by Oil of Pep-
    permint Products, Wheelton, Lancs PR6 8EP
Ortis products: distributed by Brewhurst Health Foods,
    Byfleet, Surrey
Potter's products: Herbal Supplies, Wigan
Sidroga products: Distributed by Herbalistics Ltd, Hasle-
    mere GU27 2LA
Strath products: distributed by Cedar Health Ltd, Hazel
    Grove, Cheshire SK7 5BW

Further reading

General anthroposophical and homeopathic medicine
Bott, V. *Anthroposophical Medicine. An Extension of the Art of Healing.* Steiner Press, London 1978.
—, *Spiritual Science and the Art of Healing.* Healing Arts.
Bühler, W. *Living with Your Body.* Steiner Press, London 1979.
Evans, M. *Extending the Art of Healing.* Weleda, Ilkeston.
Evans, M and I Rodger, *Healing for Body, Soul and Spirit.* Floris, Edinburgh 2000 (In America: *Complete Healing.* Anthroposophic Press, NY.
Glöckler, M. *Medicine at the Threshold of a New Consciousness.* Temple Lodge, London.
Leviton, R. *Anthroposophical Medicine Today.* Anthroposophic Press, NY.
Lockie, A. *The Family Guide to Homoeopathy.* Elm Tree, London, 1989.
Steiner, R. *Introducing Anthroposophical Medicine.* Anthroposophic Press, NY.
—, *Health and Illness.* Anthroposophic Press, NY.
—, *Overcoming Nervousness.* Anthroposophic Press, NY.
Treichler, R. *Soulways. The Developing Soul — Life Phases, Thresholds and Biography.* Hawthorn Press, Stroud 1989.
Twentyman, R. *The Science and Art of Healing.* Floris, Edinburgh.
Wolff, O. *Anthroposophically Orientated Medicine and its Remedies.* Weleda Companies.

Home nursing
Bentheim, T. van, S. Bos, E. de la Houssaye, W. Visser, *Caring for the Sick at Home.* Floris, Edinburgh, and Anthroposophic Press, NY, 1987.

Pregnancy and child care

Glas, N. *Conception, Birth and Early Childhood.* Anthroposophic Press, NY.

Glöckler, M. and W. Goebel, *A Guide to Child Health.* Floris, Edinburgh, and Anthroposophic Press, NY, 1990.

Linden, W. zur, *A Child is Born. Pregnancy, Birth, Early Childhood.* Steiner Press, London, 1980.

Salter, J. *The Incarnating Child.* Hawthorn Press, Stroud.

Creative and artistic activity

Mayer, G. *Colour and Healing.* New Knowledge Books.

Poplawski, T. *Eurythm:, Rhythm, Dance and Soul.* Floris, Edinburgh, and Anthropsophic Press, NY.

Spock, M. *Eurythmy.* Anthroposophic Press, NY.

Stebbing, L. *Music Therapy.* New Knowledge Books.

Basic nutrition and biodynamic farming

Hauschka, R. *Nutrition.* Steiner Press, London.

Koepf, H.H. *The Biodynamic Farm.* Anthroposophic Press, NY.

Schilthuis, W. *Biodynamic Agriculture.* Floris, Edinburgh, and Anthropsophic Press, NY.

Schmidt, G. *The Dynamics of Nutrition.* Biodynamic Literature.

——, *The Essentials of Nutrition.* Biodynamic Literature.

Steiner, R. *Nutrition and Health.* Anthroposophic Press, NY.

——, *Problems of Nutrition.* Anthroposophic Press, NY.

Cancer treatment

Renzenbrink, U. *Diet and Cancer.* Steiner Press, London, 1990.

Schmidt, G. *Cancer and Nutrition.* Anthroposophic Press, NY.

Cookery Book from the Lukas Clinic. Steiner Press, London.

Index